REPROGRAM
YOUR LIFE
BIOSCIENCE FOR A HEALTHIER YOU

The information contained in this book and ebook is intended to help readers make informed decisions about their health. It should not be used as a substitute for treatment by or the advice of a professional health-care provider. Follow all safety instructions before beginning any exercise or diet program. Results may vary. Exercise and proper diet are necessary to achieve and maintain a healthy lifestyle, including weight loss.

REPROGRAM YOUR LIFE:
BIOSCIENCE FOR A HEALTHIER YOU
Edited by Sheila Buff
Cover and book design by Anton Khodakovsky
Author photo by Maya Catron-Lay
Printed by BookMasters, Ashland, Ohio

First edition
GOOD HEALTH PUBLISHING

ISBN-13:
978-0-9906595-1-8

Printed in the United States of America

REPROGRAM YOUR LIFE

BIOSCIENCE FOR A HEALTHIER YOU

STEVEN WILLEY, MD

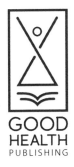

GOOD
HEALTH
PUBLISHING

Dedication

To my wonderful wife Cindy, and Jim and Mary, who have supported and encouraged me from the very beginning

TABLE OF CONTENTS

INTRODUCTION

Thousands of health-related books, products, or systems that claim to lead to good health and longevity are available right now. Each professes to be the latest breakthrough, promising to give you the results you've been longing for—better health, improved fitness, weight loss, enhanced well-being, and more energy.

Should we follow a low-fat diet, a low-carbohydrate diet, or some other type of diet? Is dairy dangerous or isn't it? Is it OK to drink diet soda or isn't it? Should we take supplements or are they a waste of money? So much information—often conflicting information—bombards us that it's virtually impossible to separate the good from the bad, the inane from the sensible, and the beneficial from the downright dangerous.

As a practicing physician, I'm constantly asked about health and fitness, including questions about diet and supplements. It seems that every few months, my patients tell me about some new "breakthrough" way to shed a few pounds. Forget about the Hollywood diet, the grapefruit diet, or the cabbage soup diet. You don't need to go to a weight-loss boot camp or have surgery. You don't need magic herbs and pills that simply don't work.

What you do need is a new approach, one that's based on a new understanding of how your body works and a new perspective on the most effective ways to reach and properly maintain your weight. This approach should include an eating plan that's simple, easy-to-follow, and based on proven research. Most important, for long-term health and vitality, the eating plan needs to be actually doable and sustainable. There's no point in losing buckets of weight on a fad diet, only to pile it all back on, with extra, when you stop. My goal in this book and with the YOU+ app and website is to help you follow a flexible, effective eating plan that leads to weight loss without deprivation or boredom.

And then there's exercise. You surely already know that exercise is good for you. But you also know that endless time on the treadmill or elliptical isn't just boring; it also isn't giving you the desired results. That same exercise time can be spent much more productively—and enjoyably—if you have a better idea of the specific types of exercise you should be doing, what order to do them in, how to vary them, and how to progress to make them really work for you. In this book and in the YOU+ app and website, I'll help you understand how often you should be exercising and for how long. I'll help you decide if interval training is the best approach for you. I'll explain about weight training and other fitness approaches, such as Pilates.

Today we're faced with so much information about exercise and fitness that we can become paralyzed by choice. Often we do nothing because we're afraid it might be the wrong thing. We're unable to commit to an approach to exercise for fear it will waste our time or lead to injury.

Those who do decide to exercise more often give up because they don't get the promised results. They get frustrated, bored, and even injured. Clearly, something is wrong with the plethora of exercise advice. Gyms across the country are full of people doing the wrong workouts the wrong way, wondering why they don't feel any better and why they don't get better results.

And that's a travesty. It's a travesty because people are investing valuable time in their health and fitness. They deserve to see great results from that commitment.

In addition, those who currently don't do any exercise look at these people and think, "It's not working for them, so why bother?" That's a travesty too, because with the right information, everyone can reap the rewards of physical exercise and fitness. No one has time for trial and error anymore. We need the definitive guide, something that works all the time, every time.

Nutrition and exercise are crucial to your health and well-being, but other aspects of your life also play an important role. Getting enough high-quality sleep and managing stress, for example, make a big difference in your ability to maintain a healthy weight and stay fit. I'll be discussing these important concepts later in this book; the YOU+ app and website help you track and improve your sleep and handle your stress, and connect them to your diet and exercise programs.

Both this book and the YOU+ app and website are your definitive lifestyle guides. This program isn't based on fad or opinion. It's an integrated approach to health, well-being, and fitness, anchored in significant scientific research and supported by serious medical expertise.

Health, well-being, and fitness can't be viewed in isolated segments. Your health isn't just about what you eat, what exercise you do, and whether you get enough sleep. It's a complex interplay among many factors in your complex life. What you do in one area of your life affects what you need to do in another. The ideal combination of diet, exercise, and sleep creates the best results. Achieving that combination is an ongoing balancing act—and the more you know, the easier it becomes to find and maintain that balance.

For example, you might not know that specific exercise techniques, combinations, order, and progressions produce significantly superior results in everything from how you look, to how much you weigh, to preventing multiple health problems. The precise techniques, combinations, order, and progressions are explained in this book and in the YOU+ app and website. They're easy to follow because they make sense and they work.

The human body is far greater than the sum of its parts. Whatever you do in one area has an effect on another area. This book and the YOU+ app and website cover all of the critical areas—nutrition, exercise, sleep, stress, and motivation—and brings them together in one integrated strategy.

Whether this program has been recommended by your forward-thinking doctor or you've found it on your own, your primary concern is, "Will it work for me?" The answer is "Yes!" But don't just take my word for it. This program works for everyone, from college students to senior citizens.

BENNETT

When Bennett left home for college at the age of 18, he was excited, but he had a hard time finding his way and dropped out after his first year. He returned home to live with his parents and started attending a local college. At 21, Bennett felt directionless, unfocused, and disorganized. Even though he exercised fairly regularly, he put on weight. Getting heavy made Bennett's self-confidence drop even more. He came to see me about his weight gain, but we ended up talking about his general sense of dissatisfaction with his life.

Bennett agreed to try the YOU+ program just to see if it would work for him. He didn't plan on doing it for a specific length of time, but his positive results came so quickly that he now plans to follow it for the long term. At the five-week mark, he had lost 18 pounds. At the ten-week mark, he had lost a total of 30 pounds. His waist circumference was down by five inches. By following the exercise program, his arms were up by half an inch and so is his chest—and he had cut 12 minutes off his 5K time. That's a significant accomplishment for someone who was simultaneously losing a substantial amount of weight. (Women follow a slightly different exercise plan and won't develop the kind increased muscle mass that Bennett did.) Because Bennett was already a fairly regular exerciser, he began the program at a relatively fit level. That makes his improvement even more remarkable and shows that proper nutrition, when combined with the proper exercises, in the right variety, order, and progression, really can make a difference.

The improvements in Bennett's fitness were matched by improvements in his mental state. He tells me that he feels more confident in all areas of his life, in everything from work and school to his relationships with the opposite sex. He says that he makes much better use of his time, is more focused and motivated, and is better primed to pursue his life goals.

MARY

Age doesn't matter when it comes to the YOU+ plan. Mary was 80 when she began to closely follow the YOU+ principles. She was overweight and out of shape—she had difficulty performing the basic activities of daily life. On the advice of her doctor, Mary decided that weight loss and fitness were worthwhile goals, even for someone of her age. Working with a trainer, Mary was diligent about her workouts—every time she set a goal of improved strength, she met it and went on to the next. In addition, by following the simple YOU+ eating plan, Mary lost a total of 63 pounds over 12 months.

At age 80, Mary could have been satisfied with enough improved strength to make a trip to the grocery store easier, but she was inspired by her own progress to go beyond that. Mary entered the Senior Olympics—and won five gold medals and one silver medal in her first attempt! She knew she could do even better, and the next year, she won eight gold medals and set three new event records.

LISA

At the age of 43, Lisa was diagnosed with high total cholesterol and triglycerides, both warning signs of heart disease to come. Although she was reasonably fit, she knew she wasn't as fit as she could be. Lisa decided to follow the YOU+ plan to improve her fitness and her diet. She worked consistently at following the principles in this book. Over the course of two years, Lisa's total cholesterol decreased from 261 to 152, her LDL cholesterol decreased from 171 to 93, and her triglycerides decreased from 166 to 72—all normal values. She feels great, looks fantastic, and is committed to the program for the long haul.

DUANE

Duane was 61 years old when he had a small stroke. At the hospital, blood tests revealed that his average blood sugar over the prior three months had been 310. Fasting blood sugar above 125 is an indicator of type 2 diabetes. Duane had been diabetic for months without knowing it; he also had high blood pressure and was overweight. As he recovered in the hospital from his stroke, a diabetes specialist suggested he start using insulin to control his blood sugar. Duane and I discussed this at length. Duane understood that without making significant lifestyle changes, he would have to spend the rest of his life injecting insulin several times a day. He convinced me that he wanted to avoid needing insulin and that he would be diligent about following the YOU+ eating plan. He wasn't kidding. A stroke and the prospect of sticking yourself with needles several times a day can be very motivating. Duane followed the eating plan carefully. He lost 40 pounds and brought down his average three-month blood sugar to 112—normal.

RUSS

Russ was a 40-something man who had done just about everything wrong when it came to health and fitness. He ate too much of the wrong things, didn't exercise, wasn't much of a sleeper, drank a bit too much, and was woefully overweight. He had reached a point in his life where he was self-conscious about his weight, and this limited his social activities and connections. He was single, lonely, and unhappy. His back hurt, his joints ached, he had high blood pressure and high blood sugar. In essence, Russ was massively shortchanging himself on life. His doctor and family had repeatedly asked him to change his ways. Despite knowing they were right, their advice seemed to go in one ear and out the other.

One day, for reasons unknown, Russ had an epiphany. He simply made up his mind that his ways really did have to change, now. Russ knew he couldn't do everything all at once, but he was eager to take incremental steps toward his goal. Working with the YOU+ principles, he started by cutting out sugared soda from his diet; he also substantially reduced processed fruit juices, substituting fresh fruit instead. He made an effort to get a protein source at every meal and cut back on unhealthy carbohydrates. Russ also decided to join a gym. He knew he needed somewhere to go so he could focus his fitness efforts. He also knew that if he stayed home, the temptation to skip exercise would be too great.

When he first met with his trainer for an initial evaluation, Russ couldn't provide an accurate weight—the scale topped out at 300 pounds, and he exceeded that. His waist was also bigger than the first tape measure used to measure him. Although flustered by these super-sized results, Russ realized that he had to start somewhere. He pushed on, joking that at least by starting from such an unhealthy position, it was going to be easy to improve. Russ started with just five minutes on the treadmill and one set of ten repetitions at a light weight for his strength training. Nothing was easy, and he didn't particularly like it, but he was persistent. Six weeks later, he was up to ten minutes on the treadmill, was able to lift somewhat heavier weights, and could do a few abdominal crunches. He had lost over two inches around his waist.

The positive results helped Russ became more focused and stick with the program. It became part of his life as the pounds continued to come off and the inches melted away. His strength, energy, stamina, and sleep improved. Most important, Russ felt like a new man. His joint pains were gone; he was off his medications for high blood pressure and high blood sugar and no longer needed anti-inflammatories for his joint pain. He became more confident, happy, and satisfied with his life, and he was last seen working out with his fiancée.

Bennett, Mary, Lisa, Duane, and Russ all embarked on a journey toward health and well-being by embracing the program detailed in this book. In doing so, they transformed their lives. What will your story be?

THE FOUNDATION

CHAPTER 1
WHY THE YOU+ METHOD WORKS

THE PRIMARY REASON THE YOU+ program works is because it applies bioscience to modern life through a new approach based on facts, medical experience, legitimate research, and results. It's not based on hype, large advertising budgets, and questionable science.

A FOUNDATION IN SCIENCE AND MEDICINE

Research and advice on fitness has typically focused on one area at a time. That area, whether the endless exercise options or nutritional and dietary recommendations, has been viewed and explored in isolation, without regard for the fact that how and what you do in one area affects what you need to do in other areas of your health. The YOU+ method incorporates the latest serious, research-based information on what modern science has shown is safe, effective, and good for your health.

The substantial shift in research dogma in recent years shouldn't really come as a big surprise. After all, if what we thought we knew was so effective, then we would all be super-fit and healthy from following programs based on those principles we thought were right. The reality, however, is quite different. As a nation, our overall physical condition and health has steadily deteriorated. For the first time since the Civil War, the lifespan of Americans is expected to decrease in the twenty-first century. You can confidently expect to live longer than your great-grandparents did, but your children may well die at a younger age than you. This is a complicated issue, but clearly, what we think we know doesn't work. Up until now, we haven't yet found a consistently doable and effective formula to health, wellbeing, and fitness.

The YOU+ program changes that. The information you'll learn from me has been exhaustively researched and proven. It's based on careful studies that have been reported in reliable scientific journals. It has also been thoroughly vetted and fine-tuned through my extensive personal experience with my patients. In the upcoming chapters, you'll gain a working understanding of the basic principles of the YOU+ method. I'll help you learn how to separate true from false and effective from noneffective. YOU+ brings together a vast amount of information from a wide range of reputable scientific sources and puts it into a coherent, practical system you can easily understand—and easily follow. Much of what you will learn is a new paradigm approach to fitness and health. It's different from what you may have read or tried, but it works. And you can take that to the bank!

Do you remember the 1973 Woody Allen movie *Sleeper?* In it, the protagonist is cryogenically frozen for two hundred years and then revived in a futuristic society. Among the things he discovers is that many of the practices thought healthful in his lifetime were, in fact, just the opposite. While the story line is fictional, the concept is not. Just think of smoking. There was a time, several decades ago, when people—even doctors—genuinely believed that smoking wasn't physically harmful, and yet today, that idea seems utterly absurd. The same is true of many of the health "facts" we currently believe to be true. Often, when researchers look carefully at the conventional wisdom, it turns out to be incorrect. For example, many nutritionists tell their overweight clients to eat smaller, more frequent meals, saying this will raise their metabolism and speed up weight loss. In fact, recent research shows the opposite to be true.

It's time to sweep out the old and make way for the new so we can achieve good health without the confusion. The YOU+ method wipes away lingering misconceptions and integrates proven new findings into your fitness plan. This fresh approach gives you a clear path to achieving your health and fitness goals.

That research has generally focused on one area of fitness in isolation and not in relation to others has also held back progress. Typically, studies have focused on diet, exercise, sleep, or stress in and of themselves, but not on the factors that determine how they interrelate. This is finally beginning to change. We now have a much better understanding of what happens when we combine these factors and look at how the they interact. In some ways, this singular focus on just one health aspect and the lack of understanding regarding interdependence among all the factors acts like sweeping a mess under the rug. On the surface, you appear to have solved a problem and to have done a good thing, but all you've really done is to shift the problem to another realm. No real, long-lasting result is achieved. You haven't eliminated the mess; you've simply moved it somewhere else to create different problems. The same goes for fitness and health. If you aren't combining the right type of diet with the right type and amount of exercise, the right nutrition, and the right quality of sleep, you won't achieve the results you hoped for. And let's face it—most of us don't have much spare time. Who has the time for trial-and-error health and fitness? What we all want is a proven, definitive guide on what to do. We want the time and effort we invest to pay real dividends. My goal in YOU+ is to clarify all of this for you so you will know how to get the most out of what you do and the time and effort you put in. Why waste your time on anything else?

The YOU+ method takes the smart approach to fitness. It's designed to make your investment of time and effort pay maximum dividends. This book gives you a solid grasp of the basic YOU+ method, but to keep the program at the cutting edge, I also strongly recommend using the YOU+ website and app.

Research on human health is ongoing. YOU+ tracks the steady stream of new discoveries in many different areas and constantly refines current thinking on techniques for fitness and health. The website and app provide a weekly plan to follow for optimal results, while weaving the latest actionable, peer-reviewed discoveries into the program so that it's always up-to-date. YOU+ provides the information and tools you need to take charge of your life and your health in a positive way.

THE FOUR YOU+ PRINCIPLES

Four key principles are fundamental to why the YOU+ program works:

1. Insulin efficiency

2. Gastrointestinal hormones

3. The opposing forces of breakdown and repair

4. Nutrient timing

In the rest of this book, I'll explain why understanding each principle is indispensable for helping you to appreciate the rationale for your fitness and health plan. The YOU+ program outlined in this book will help you support your body back into healthy balance so it can do what it does best. I want to empower you to own your health and well-being once and for all. This is, after all, *your* YOU+, and it is *your* gateway to health.

INSULIN EFFICIENCY

The hormone insulin, produced in your pancreas, plays a central role in your body. Insulin is responsible for carrying glucose (blood sugar), your body's primary source of fuel, into your cells, where it is burned for energy. Without insulin, you would die.

Insulin is also the hormone your body uses to store fat. After insulin carries enough glucose into your cells to meet their needs, it takes whatever glucose is left over and carries it off to be stored as fat.

For peak health and fitness, the insulin you produce needs to be used efficiently. To use your insulin efficiently, you want to produce just enough of it to meet your metabolic needs—and no more. Ironically, most of us can't use our insulin efficiently because we produce too much of it.

Here's how it works. As you put on those extra pounds, or even just as you get older, your cells become resistant to the effect of insulin. Your pancreas has to produce more of it just to force enough glucose into your cells. Your blood sugar values are still in the normal range, so it appears that everything is fine, but you're now making a lot more insulin to keep those numbers within normal limits. You don't have type 2 diabetes (insulin resistance so bad that your blood sugar is high all the time), at least not yet. What you do have is a lot of extra insulin sloshing around in your bloodstream.

Whether or not you're insulin resistant, keeping your insulin levels as low as possible—using your insulin efficiently—is crucial for reaching your health and fitness goals.

Insulin resistance and the resultant increased insulin levels can lead to a cascade of devastating effects, including weight gain, cancer, high blood pressure, heart disease, stroke, kidney disease, dementia, and diminished quality of life. These outcomes aren't in question; the medical evidence is irrefutable. Insulin resistance will absolutely keep you from meeting your health, fitness, and weight goals, and it will continue to impact your results until you do something about it. The majority of the concepts discussed in this book are designed to create insulin efficiency and reduce the negative impacts of insulin resistance.

The idea of evaluating specific exercise techniques and dietary changes in the context of insulin efficiency is a new and very powerful framework. The YOU+ method is unique in using these groundbreaking new concepts as its foundation.

INSULIN EFFICIENCY EXPLAINED

Let's take a closer look at insulin. You may think of it as something only people with diabetes need to think about. In fact, however, insulin is crucial to all of us, because it controls our blood sugar levels and our body fat. Insulin's primary job is as an energy storage hormone. When we eat something, our blood glucose level increases, signaling the pancreas to release insulin to use it. The insulin then does its job. Some of the glucose is carried to your body's cells to be used for energy; some is carried to your liver to be stored as glycogen, the body's go-to source of quick energy. The rest is carried off to be converted to fat, your body's way to store the energy for later use.

Without insulin, you can't store fat. The more insulin, the more fat storage. When insulin levels drop, the reverse happens—energy stored as fat is utilized and burned. The important thing to know is that the less excess insulin you have floating around, the better off you are going to be. Sounds pretty simple, right?

It's actually not that simple at all. In fact, it's extraordinarily complex. Because energy storage is so important to the survival of the species, your body has multiple pathways involved in energy storage and burning. Energy storage and use are based not only on what you eat but also on the exercise you do and the sleep you get.

A tiny part of the brain called the hypothalamus has a huge say in what happens. The hypothalamus receives signals from many parts of the body, including those that tell it whether you're hungry or full. It also gets signals about your general degree of fat storage. All of that information reaching the hypothalamus triggers signals in return. The hypothalamus sends messages to the body, telling you if you should eat or not and if you should feel energetic or not.

An extremely important signal to the hypothalamus comes from the hormone leptin. Leptin is made by fat cells. If you have a lot of fat cells, you make a lot of leptin. A high leptin level tells the hypothalamus that you now have plenty of stored energy and don't need to eat to get more fuel. In fact, it's now OK to feel like being active and have a sense of well-being. But this is where the plot thickens.

High insulin levels block the leptin signal from working in the hypothalamus. Even if you're overweight from too much stored energy and are producing a lot of leptin from all that extra fat, your hypothalamus isn't getting the message. It thinks your energy balance is too low (you're starving) and tells your body to do whatever it can to *increase* energy stores. In other words, you feel hungry and less energetic because your hypothalamus is telling you to eat more and conserve energy.

Remember, insulin resistance means you need higher levels of insulin to get the job done. But insulin resistance also means more insulin in your bloodstream, which blocks the leptin signal and causes a cascade of overeating, underexercising, and all the negative things that come from that. When you improve insulin efficiency, your insulin levels are lower, leptin isn't blocked, and your hypothalamus gets the leptin message clearly. You feel better, look better, and are far healthier.

The insulin/leptin connection doesn't stop at the hypothalamus. Another brain pathway that is affected by insulin and leptin is the one that regulates "reward." In other words, this brain function, also known as the dopamine pathway, makes you feel good in response to something. Most researchers believe the pathway is there to make sure behaviors that are important to survival of the species are desirable and produce a positive feeling of reward. Sex is pleasurable, so we want to do it, thereby ensuring reproduction. Food is pleasurable, so we want to eat it, thus getting the nutrition necessary to live. The reward pathways are particularly strong for foods that are palatable, meaning they're high in sugar and fat.

As you might imagine, the reward system in your brain is highly complex. What's relevant to us, however, is that leptin helps extinguish the feeling of reward from food. When leptin levels are high because you have enough body fat, the reward pathway becomes less responsive. That lowers your desire for food because you don't get as much of a reward from eating— it becomes less pleasurable. You eat less and put your energy toward other things.

Guess what too much insulin does to the dopamine reward pathway? You're right—the increased insulin levels from insulin resistance keeps leptin from acting appropriately. When insulin blocks leptin's actions in the reward pathway, you continue to get increased pleasure from your food, even though you don't need to eat more for energy. In other words, you don't feel satiated by your food, even when you eat a lot of it. Over time, it takes even more of those sweet and fatty foods to give you the same satisfaction that you got in the beginning.

This leads to our eating more and more and creates pleasure when we do. Now you know why you crave all of those things that you know just aren't good for you. Think about it. When your insulin efficiency is poor—or, in other words, when your insulin levels are higher than they need to be—the signals that tell you to stop eating are blurred. Your body tells you that you need to eat more, even when you don't. It tells you that you're tired and need to conserve energy, even when you don't need to, so you feel less like being active and have a lowered sense of well-being. And your body tells you that sugary and fatty foods sure look good. It's no wonder the Twinkie was so popular that they had to bring it back after it was discontinued. And it's no wonder we can't stick to an eating program and have success.

That's why the YOU+ program works. It's specifically designed to improve insulin efficiency and lower insulin resistance and insulin levels. When that happens, your body sends the right signals at the right time—and the signals get through as they should. If you've tried other approaches, that's why they haven't worked out over the long term. They didn't deal with the fundamental underlying issue of insulin resistance and didn't restore your insulin efficiency.

If you have all of these factors constantly fighting against you, it creates a tremendous headwind to success. In this book and with the YOU+ app and website, I give you all the tools you need to put the wind at your back. The type, variety, order, and progression of exercise is vital to improving insulin efficiency. If you aren't doing this the right way, you aren't going to get much bang for the buck. The proper nutritional strategy is of course another key. And knowing the proper approach to sleep helps you even more—the quality of your sleep has surprisingly far-reaching effects on your health. Any one of these components is helpful, but optimal health is definitely a case where the whole is greater than the sum of the parts.

The YOU+ method takes into account how these factors interrelate. By combining them all in an intelligent way, you will reap tremendous rewards. This is a battle that can be won so long as you know you're *in* a battle and you understand the right way to fight.

GASTROINTESTINAL HORMONES

The study of gastrointestinal hormones—the hormones produced by the stomach and intestines—has turned into a very exciting area of research. As you now know, the system regulating your weight and its subsequent health effects is far more complicated than we once thought. It's an intertwining system that involves complex feedback and feed-forward loops among your gut, your fat cells, and your brain.

Let's explore how the actions of the hormones produced by your gastrointestinal tract play an important and active role in the signals that regulate your weight and health.

Dozens of the many natural chemicals produced by your gastrointestinal tract can potentially help you reach, or keep you from reaching, your health goals. They have weird names like peptide YY, ghrelin, and CCK. You don't need to know all the details about how they work, but understanding the basics of a few of the most important hormones will give you what you need to know.

Peptide YY (also known as pancreatic peptide YY 3–36—see what I mean about details?) is produced by your small intestine. When you eat a meal, especially a meal that has fat and protein in it, peptide YY is released into your bloodstream and carried to your brain. It is one of the pathways that tells your brain you're full and don't need to eat any more. Peptide YY also works within the digestive tract by slowing down the speed of the digestive process. Again, that makes you feel full and acts as a signal to stop eating.

Does this sound familiar? Like leptin, peptide YY works through the hypothalamus and the reward pathways to promote changes that make you feel more satisfied by your food. You therefore eat less while, importantly, feeling less hungry.

The hormone ghrelin, produced by cells in the lining of your stomach, is responsible for making you feel hungry. (It also stimulates the release of growth hormone, something I'll discuss more in the chapter on the importance of sleep.) When your stomach is empty, ghrelin is released and sends a message to the brain saying you're hungry. When your stomach is full, ghrelin release ceases, and you stop feeling hungry. Not all of your gastrointestinal hormones act primarily by being messengers to your brain. Incretins, another type of gastrointestinal hormone, directly affect the all-important insulin system. Two types of incretin hormones are of particular interest to us. They have long names that we can conveniently shorten to GLP-1 and GIP. These two incretins are secreted only in response to food. They send signals to your pancreas to release insulin into your bloodstream in advance of the rise in blood sugar that will happen later, as the glucose from your food is absorbed. This actually helps lower your blood sugar after a meal.

Incretins also slow the emptying of your stomach so nutrient absorption is more efficient. When your stomach empties more slowly, you feel full sooner and for longer, and your blood sugar doesn't spike up as much, which in turn means that you don't need to pump out as much insulin to carry the blood sugar away. Because you want to keep your insulin level down, you can see why this is so helpful. As you might expect, having good levels of incretin hormones has been proven to lead to weight loss.

What if you could harness the power of your gastrointestinal tract hormones to your advantage? You can, and that is exactly what the YOU+ nutritional plan does. You'll learn what and when to eat to get the most out of these advantages. And best of all, you'll learn how to succeed without starving yourself or counting calories.

OPTIMIZING THE FORCES OF BREAKDOWN AND REPAIR

Your body isn't a machine that always stays the same. You have constant turnover in your cells—constant breakdown and repair, out with the old and in with the new. You don't have exactly the same cells in your body that you had yesterday, let alone six months ago.

This process is carried out by opposing systems in the body. One system breaks things down, and another system builds things back up once the breakdown has been cleared. These processes involve hundreds of body chemicals and are highly intricate and complicated. For example, certain natural chemicals can sometimes be used for breakdown, and the same chemicals can also be used for building things back up. It's important to remember that these opposing processes are supposed to happen. Your body needs both opposing forces as a way to constantly repair itself and keep from becoming worn out at the cellular level.

If your body were a house, think of it as the carpet getting overly worn. Your body fixes the problem by sending the breakdown team to tear out the old, worn carpet. The repair team then comes in and lays the new replacement carpet. The system isn't always quite as neat and straightforward. The processes that promote breakdown actually cause more damage than was present initially. It's as if the breakdown team comes into your house, spills grape juice all over the carpet, and uses sharp objects to poke holes in it, just to make sure the carpet is really in need of repair. This "over the top" breakdown system has a purpose, however, and achieves something very helpful. The breakdown team's presence on site automatically informs the carpet layers that they need to come and fix the carpet. They give directions on how to get there and tell them the extent of the repair work needed. The carpet layers come, do their job, and the next thing you know, your house has carpet that's as good as new.

The critical point here is that the breakdown team calls in the repair team. It takes damage to trigger repair, and damage is necessary to cause the signal for that repair to take place. The same thing happens in your body, but here, the damage is called inflammation. Some level of inflammation is part of the healing and renewal process and is necessary to signal the body to repair itself. The chemicals themselves involved in the inflammation give the signal for repair and renewal.

When the opposing systems are out of balance, there's more breakdown than repair. The result is disease. As we get older, the balance naturally shifts toward breakdown over repair. Even so, we can shift the balance back in our favor. The YOU+ program helps your body to use its own opposing systems to your advantage. I'll show you how.

DIETARY SUPPLEMENTS AND NUTRIENT TIMING

How and when to take dietary supplements is an area that is rarely spoken about in the medical office. Substantial and credible literature validates the use of a very limited number of supplements to improve the results from your fitness efforts. Some of the supplements I'll discuss here aren't part of standard medical advice, simply because this is an area where the connection between the data and the general health of the population is unrecognized and undervalued in the current priorities of the health-care system.

The key, however, is in knowing not only which supplements have value but also in knowing exactly when and how these should be taken. If this isn't done correctly, you might as well throw your money away, rather than spend it on useless supplements. The type and intensity of your exercise program will dictate what supplements you take and when you take them. The interrelationship between nutrient timing and exercise isn't usually fully understood by most medical professionals, let alone the general population. This is no wonder, given the plethora of supplement products on the market, each making a different claim. Telling truth from fiction and marketing is impossible without a careful study of the experimental evidence.

That's where the YOU+ method comes in. I've studied that evidence and combined it with my experience as both a practicing physician and someone who works out regularly. I'll explain exactly what you need to know to take full advantage of this important aspect of health and fitness. The nutrients we'll discuss are naturally found in our diet. The amounts needed are normally achievable, so the trick is simply to know how to isolate them, when to take them, and how much to take to get the most benefit. But before we get to that, let me give you some pointers on how to navigate the jungle of fact and fiction known as wellness.

CHAPTER 2
WELLNESS

WELLNESS IS A TERM that has lost its way. While well-intentioned, wellness has come to symbolize a broad-brush definition of health. The term is now so widely used that it has clouded our ability to learn the truth about what is truly beneficial to our health and well-being. Let's take a look at how to evaluate health and fitness information so you can get your personal wellness back on track.

Improvements in your lifestyle and personal wellness won't come about by magic. They come from a true inner desire to better your life and to meet your full potential, whatever your age. You have to want it. What do you want to accomplish? How is your current lifestyle working for you?

I want you to feel better *now*. I want you to look the way you want to look, while also reducing your risk of disease. If you can do that, then you increase your chances for a high-quality life—a life that is not just long but full and fun. There is no point in growing older and just existing. Let's be real: we're all going to die of something, but not everyone truly lives.

The adjustments you make to your lifestyle need to be the *right* adjustments; otherwise, you are wasting your precious time and resources. This chapter will help you understand what a right adjustment is and how it can help.

SCIENCE (FICTION) OR SCIENCE (FACT)

To make those right adjustments, you must follow principles based on real, validated science—not an exaggeration or distortion of science; not a fad, a fiction, or hearsay. You must be able to trust the source of your information. As simple as that sounds, it's not always easy. For starters, our cultural expectation and understanding of wellness has been corrupted. Wellness has become a highly lucrative business. A business needs to make a profit, and a profit requires sales. More and bigger sales require more new products and services and more new ways to sell them. This endless demand for bigger profits has caused a huge disconnect in the wellness industry. Many wellness products and programs are useful, but the drive for profit has created countless shams and scams. Distorted or outright false information and faulty, disconnected "science" full of half-truths and misconceptions have come to dominate the wellness industry. The American public is bombarded with products that promise fast, easy answers, such as killer abs in three minutes a day or quick weight loss through one weird trick. When profit is the primary motivation, genuine wellness is left behind as people spend vast amounts of money on products that provide short-lived hope but little else.

What most people don't realize is that the great majority of these products are not regulated by the Food and Drug Administration (FDA). Products with claims that say *maintain, support,* or *promote* don't need to have any proof whatsoever. This is true whether you buy them on the Internet or at a major national retailer. Nonetheless, a recent consumer survey revealed that more than half of the survey respondents believed that these product claims were regulated by the FDA. Even worse, more than 60 percent falsely believed that these types of products had been tested and found to be safe and effective.

I was recently at a health exposition that featured hundreds of products related to fitness. I observed a man talking to a sales rep about a particular product. As a doctor, I could tell the product claims didn't really fit with what it could realistically do. Nevertheless, the rep made a sale. After the customer walked away with his bag, the sales rep said to another rep, "I love America. You can sell anything!"

The claims for the efficacy of many supplements and other health-related products are often based on "scientific" studies that supposedly support the product. In advertisements, you'll often see images of scientists in pristine white lab coats or other images meant to convey an authoritative and trustworthy impression. The reality is that many of these "scientific" studies wouldn't be accepted at my kid's junior high science fair. The product studies are generally done for marketing purposes, not science. If you look at the annual reports of the many unregulated companies in this "profit over substance" sector, you'll often see that two-thirds of their budget is spent on marketing. Only about 5 percent of their budget is spent on actual research and development. Contrast that to the regulated pharmaceutical and device companies that must meet very high standards of evidence for the efficacy and safety of their products. These companies spend 20 to 30 percent of their budget on research and development. Doesn't this show where the emphasis really is?

When wellness is a business, it's difficult to separate fact from fiction. Consider the use of the word "natural" in advertising. Most people assume natural is also good, and I agree that natural is usually a desirable characteristic. But simply because something is natural doesn't mean it is effective or even safe. We still want to see some evidence that shows it's safe and actually does something positive for your health.

Among consumers, and even among health professionals who should know better, there's a pervasive belief that a natural substance is safe even when it's taken in concentrated form or in large doses. I had a patient call me one night with what sounded like a significant allergic reaction. We went through her exposures that day to figure out what the reaction could be from. She mentioned she had received an injection from another provider. When I asked her if she had talked to him about her reaction, she said she had. He told her it couldn't be a reaction to the injection, because what he injected was natural. That's like saying you couldn't have a reaction to a bee sting because, of course, that's natural.

If health providers are willing to say things like that to promote their practice, it's no wonder that marketers will, too. You've probably seen ads claiming that because the product, whatever it is, is all natural, it doesn't have any side effects. In reality, if the product really has any effect, then by definition it has the potential for a side effect. You can't have one without the chance for the other. The only way to truly claim a product doesn't have potential for a side effect is if it doesn't have any effect at all. And if it has no effect at all, then why would you take it?

A natural product isn't necessarily a safe one. Hemlock is natural—but that won't stop it from killing you! Tobacco is natural—and it will kill you too, though more slowly than hemlock. Taking too much all-natural vitamin C will upset your digestion just as much as taking too much of the synthetic version.

Another favorite trick of the wellness industry is to exaggerate a claim that stems from a basic scientific truth. When a particular substance is known to have a function in the body, supplement manufacturers use that to make that claim that taking more of it must promote more of that function. If an enzyme you naturally make in your cells is involved in the pathways that produce energy in the body, for example, supplement manufacturers claim that taking it in their pills will surely improve your energy even further. Saying A is good so more of A will be better is a mental leap that rarely has any merit. It's like saying that if two aspirin are good for a headache, then twenty must be great. Another pitfall of these product claims is that the product you swallow may not end up in your body in the same form. When something is actually made in the body, it goes straight into your bloodstream—it doesn't go through the digestive process. A supplement, on the other hand, does. Your body digests the supplement and may break it down into smaller parts. If the supposed effect comes only when the product is still in the whole form, and not in digested fragments, it will do nothing. Even if it is absorbed whole through the small intestine, it must then pass through the liver, where it may well be broken down before entering the main blood supply. Many products don't survive this process and end up being less effective than claimed, or not effective at all.

Many of the "scientific" studies used for product claims and promotion are sponsored by the company itself. Others are sponsored by an "institute" or some other organization that is affiliated with the company. How reliable is it when a nutritional company researches itself? In a recent article about sports nutrition and weight loss products, the *National Business Journal* lists "in-house publishing" as the first approach under the heading, "Strategies of Sports Nutrition and Weight Loss Marketers." Many wellness promoters lure people to websites designed to look like independent news sources that indirectly recommend the promoters' supplements or other products. This isn't very comforting.

WELLNESS CENTERS OR PROFIT CENTERS?

Wellness centers seem to be popping up all over the place to try to address the need for health guidance.

Anything that increases overall wellness is certainly welcome, but unfortunately, this is an area that is almost completely unregulated. Consumers have no way of knowing if the people providing advice, products, and services at a wellness center are qualified to do so. Just as you can't take advertisers' claims at face value, you should never assume expertise based on anything other than solid, verifiable proof and genuine credentials. Just because someone wears a white coat he bought on eBay doesn't make him a doctor. Just because there are ornate certificates in expensive frames on the wall from such-and-such an institute doesn't make him an expert. When you realize that many of these "institutes" basically sell their certification to anyone who pays their fees to take their online "training," you realize that they are nothing but profit-making businesses. Many of their "graduates" know little about health or nutrition, but they know a lot about persuading you to buy their services and products. The same is true of supplement stores that have their employees take a course to become "certified." The employees are being certified not in nutrition but in ways to sell you supplements. I recently saw a storefront sign that advertised "Hair, Nails, and Weight Loss." That's a little like advertising your services as biologist, geneticist, and pastry chef! In truth, I don't know anything about that particular proprietor, but I do know that the science of weight loss is an extremely complex area that is very different from hair and nails. Bet your well-being only on practitioners who have genuine training that can be verified.

Some of the many wellness centers now operating across the country offer "tests" that claim to determine your state of wellness and discover any deficiencies you may have. Then, lo and behold, you just happen to have the deficiency they tested you for, and they just happen to sell a supplement or treatment that's the cure. Doesn't it seem odd that they just happen to sell what they claim you need? That they just happen to focus your testing on areas in which they carry products? This is not to say the proprietors don't truly believe what they are doing is sound. That belief, however, doesn't make up for their shortcomings. Their evaluations aren't at all the same thing as a comprehensive medical history and exam done by a trained and experienced medical practitioner. Their evaluations and treatments are often based on poor or distorted science.

SEPARATING FACT FROM FICTION

My patients often ask me how they can tell the difference between a study that was done for marketing purposes and one that was done using valid, verifiable science. One way is to see if the study was controlled. A controlled study compares groups of people who are similar in important characteristics, such as gender, age, smoking history, exercise history, or the presence of a particular medical problem. Comparing the effects of a supplement on a group of nursing home residents to a group of 25-year-old fitness enthusiasts isn't controlled—the results wouldn't be valid. Likewise, it's not valid to compare overweight swimmers who smoke to underweight nonsmokers who don't exercise. The examples I've given are obvious, but it's easy to manipulate even subtle differences in groups to increase the chances of getting the result you want.

The sizes of the groups compared can also lead to skewed results. The larger the group the less likely something will occur by chance. If you flip a coin four times and get heads three times, you could say your method of coin flipping resulted in heads 75 percent of the time. Technically, that's true. But does it reflect reality? If you flip a coin a hundred times, it is much harder to defy the 50–50 odds. It's the same principle casinos use. The casino has only a slight edge in the odds, but over large volumes of activity, they invariably come out ahead. They don't build those lavish properties in Las Vegas by losing!

The same principle applies to small study groups. If you compare two groups of ten people, and in one group four get a particular result and in the other group five get a particular result, you could claim the second group had a 25 percent greater response to whatever is being tested. If you were a supplement marketer, you would then plaster this all over your promotional material, claiming it was proven in a "scientific study." Was it? No. With such small numbers, the difference in the result could easily have been due to chance, just like getting three heads in four coin flips. Marketers have a strong incentive to create, select, and promote trials that give them the greatest amount of profit. Is that the way you should make choices on something as important as your health? Sadly, many people do, but you don't need to. That's what this book, the YOU+ app, and the website are for: to help you make the best choices based on the best and most current scientific information.

All of the research and scientific studies cited in this book, in the YOU+ app, and on the website are valid, verifiable, and controlled. The research is published in respected, peer-reviewed scientific and medical journals. The results aren't manipulated to fit a hypothesis or fulfill a marketing brief. Whether you're reading this book because it was recommended to you by your forward-thinking doctor or because you came across it on your own, what you will learn here will help you finally achieve true fitness and wellness.

SECTION 2
NUTRITION

CHAPTER 3
WHAT TO EAT AND WHY

I AM ALWAYS UP front and completely honest with my patients, so I'm going to be the same way in this book. I believe that eating is one of the greatest physical pleasures in life. Only a small minority of people will be able to stick with a dietary plan that takes away that pleasure for any length of time. Food should not be looked at as medicine, with the sole purpose of providing some sort of nutritional benefit. Food is a way to indulge your senses. Food is fun; sharing meals with family and friends is a wonderful way to bond.

If you're knowledgeable, eating can still give you that pleasure while also meeting your body's requirements for optimal health. I promise you—good food and good health can coexist. You may have to revise the way you look at some foods, and getting results may take some time, but I can tell you without doubt that changing your approach to your diet for the better can happen for you.

From the start, I want to be clear about your own expectations. It's unreasonable to think that you'll be perfect all the time. You're going to eat things that you know aren't good for you—I do. Thinking that you'll eat exactly as you should from now on is an unrealistic expectation that only sets you up for a cycle of guilt. Everyone has days or longer periods where they make unhealthy choices, despite their best efforts. In fact, these aberrations are probably necessary for the majority of us to stay on track for the long run. We're not robots, and we can't be expected to be programmed the way they are. The key here is that unhealthy choices need to be the exception, not the normal mode of operation. That expectation is reasonable and achievable.

The need for an occasional dietary indiscretion reminds me of a family wedding I attended in San Francisco. My wife, kids, and I were in town for the event, along with many other family members, some of whom we hadn't seen for quite some time. Conversations naturally included what everyone was doing at the time. When asked, I was enthusiastic about my area of specialization and the experiences I have had helping patients with fitness.

The events of the day unfolded, and we had just returned from a fairly late evening. My wife and kids were going to bed. The hotel was near a marina and the weather was nice, so I decided to take a brief walk. As I rounded the first corner, the air was thick with the delicious smell of freshly cooked doughnuts. It was impossible to ignore its presence in the cool night air. I walked over to the small shop and peered through the glass. A few minutes later, I walked out with a glazed old-fashioned doughnut in my hand. Never mind that it was about as unhealthy as it gets—fried white flour made with white sugar. It was also after midnight, I was alone on a walk, and who was going to see me? As I put the doughnut in my mouth for the first bite, the silence of the evening was shattered by "Steve, are you still up?" It was a group of my wife's aunts and cousins. I'd been caught red-handed! Looking at me and then the doughnut, one of them smiled and said, "Aren't you supposed to be Dr. Fitness or something?"

I confess it wasn't my finest professional moment, but it was an important reminder of realistic expectations and looking at the big picture. If you do things right consistently, you have room for indulgences now and then—even unhealthy, dough-nut-shaped indulgences. Doing things the right way should, however, still be enjoyable—otherwise it's unsustainable over the long term. A healthy approach can still taste great.

In America, it seems that we just aren't getting this right. The number of overweight and obese people has been climb-ing steadily. In fact, almost one-third of our population is obese, meaning their body weight is 20 percent more than is con-sidered healthy for their height. If we include people who are overweight, nearly two-thirds of the population is carrying an unhealthy amount of extra weight. This is taking its toll on all of us as health-care costs skyrocket.

Insulin resistance is a major factor in why our calorie intakes are up and our activity levels are down. When you don't use insulin efficiently, the extra that floats around in your blood has a major impact on your appetite, your activity level, and your will power. The bottom line? We're all responsible for our own actions. Are you going to take action to make sure your body uses insulin as efficiently as it should? Ultimately, we decide for ourselves if we win or lose the health battle.

Recently, some researchers have argued that the dangers of being overweight are overstated. In a good example of how "evi-dence" can be misinterpreted or manipulated, this assertion is based on studies that compared groups of people who were all overweight to groups that included everyone else. The problem, however, was that the mixed groups included not only people who were normal weight but also those who were underweight, presumably due to already existing health conditions. This skewed the findings, because most of the underweight people were probably too thin because they had a serious underlying health problem. By comparison, the groups of overweight people seemed healthier than they actually were. The only valid study is to compare a group of people who are all of healthy weight to a group of people who are all overweight. Whenever this is done, the health ramifications of being overweight are impossible to ignore.

TRUTH AND CONSEQUENCES

Substantial research on the health impacts of being overweight or obese shows some alarming trends. For example, if you're overweight but not obese, you are up to 40 percent more likely to die prematurely of any cause. This can be true even if you consider yourself healthy except for your weight. In a Northwestern University study that followed more than 17,000 people for 30 years, being overweight in midlife increased the risk of dying from heart disease later, even among participants who had normal blood pressure and cholesterol at the start of the study. This is counter to the common but misguided perception that being overweight isn't a problem until or unless your blood pressure and cholesterol levels also increase.

We know that being overweight increases your risk of cancer and diabetes. According to the World Cancer Research Fund, 340,000 cases of cancer can be prevented each year in the United States just by modifying diet, exercise, and alcohol intake. That is a huge number and doesn't even include smoking-related cancers.

Being overweight has more immediate and obvious consequences as well: back pain, knee pain, lack of energy and vigor, and a good chance of erectile dysfunction in men.

Being overweight in midlife is also a risk factor for Alzheimer's disease. The extra weight can cause deterioration in your memory later, and there is evidence it can affect your memory *now*. Research from the Women's Health Initiative, a long-term, multicenter trial that tracked more than 160,000 older women for over 15 years starting in 1991 found that for every 1 point increase in body mass index (a standard measure for body weight), there was a 1 point drop in cognitive performance scores. This association persisted even after controlling for high blood pressure and diabetes, which suggests that the loss of cognitive ability isn't just from poor blood circulation to the brain. The researchers felt that being overweight, in and of itself, was probably affecting the brain.

Another study, published in the respected journal *Human Brain Mapping* in 2009, used brain imaging to show that brains of obese people had 8 percent less brain tissue and appeared 16 years older than the brains of lean individuals. Those who were merely overweight had 4 percent less brain tissue and brains that appeared 8 years older than lean individuals.

METABOLIC SYNDROME

The rise in weight has paralleled the rise in a collection of health risk factors known as the metabolic syndrome. Remember how earlier I talked about the cascade of changes in our hormones, brains, weight, and general health that result from the mere presence of insulin resistance? And how important it is to use insulin efficiently, even if your weight is normal and you don't have insulin resistance? The metabolic syndrome, a group of risk factors that sharply increases your chances for type 2 diabetes, heart disease, stroke, circulatory problems, and other life-threatening health conditions, is a dangerous step in the progression toward worsening health. The lack of insulin efficiency and excess weight that are hallmarks of the metabolic syndrome are also associated with cancer and Alzheimer's disease. Plus, you simply won't feel (or look) as good as you could.

The metabolic syndrome isn't a disease in itself. Instead, it's a set of markers that warn of the strong likelihood of disease, both now and in the future. Nearly 25 percent of the adult population in the United States already have the metabolic syndrome. Of individuals age 50 and older, about 40 percent have it.

To find out if you already have the metabolic syndrome, answer the following questions:

Do you have a waist circumference of 40 inches or more for men or 35 inches or more for women?	**Yes**	**No**

Note: *This is not your pant size, which can run 2 inches larger or lower than your real waist measurement. Use a tape measure to find your true waist measurement.*

Is your blood pressure 130/85 or higher, or are you taking blood pressure medication?	**Yes**	**No**

Is your triglyceride level above 150 mg/dl?	**Yes**	**No**

Is your fasting blood sugar level above 100 mg/dl, or are you taking blood sugar lowering medication?	**Yes**	**No**

Is your HDL cholesterol level below 40mg/dl for men or below 50 mg/dl for women?	**Yes**	**No**

If you answered yes to three or more of these questions, then you not only have insulin resistance, which in and of itself is harmful, but you also have already progressed to the full-blown metabolic syndrome.

Don't panic. You can still turn your health around.

In this book, with the YOU+ app, and on the website, you'll learn the ideal nutritional strategy for making your insulin use more efficient and reversing the metabolic syndrome. You'll learn about the type, variety, order, and progression of exercise that will help, along with other important components that will not only help you to cure or prevent insulin resistance but also prevent the progression to the full-blown metabolic syndrome and the health conditions it can bring. This is the knowledge you need to help you get control of your health so you can feel and look your best.

The metabolic syndrome is now so widespread that conflicting and false information about how to handle it abounds. It's almost impossible to sort out what's good advice and what's bad, much less figure out what to do to achieve the best results. Often the information is conflicting; one report claims that a certain food or drink is good for you, while another says it's bad. You might well feel overwhelmed by the sheer volume of conflicting information.

To help you see the truth through the confusion, in this book, in the YOU+ app, and on the website, I give you only the information you *need* to understand insulin efficiency and how to fix the metabolic syndrome. My goal is to help you appreciate what you need to do and why.

Following a plan is always much easier when you truly understand why it works as effectively as it does. It's also easier to follow that plan when you fully appreciate the consequences and ramifications for your health when you don't.

UNDERSTANDING YOUR FOOD

To make sense of the YOU+ program, we need to take a look at the components that make up your food: the various types of fats, carbohydrates, and protein. Although many health-care professionals still stick to outdated ideas about nutrition, the dogma is clearly beginning to change. In this section, I'll remove the myths and the hype to give you definitive information about food and nutrition. What you learn here is backed by research, science, clinical trials, and my practical experience with my patients—not a big marketing budget. And after you've learned it, you'll be able to incorporate that knowledge into a plan that will be simple to incorporate into your life.

Let's start by exploring the truth about:

- Saturated fat
- Dairy foods
- Red meat
- Polyunsaturated fats
- Monounsaturated fat
- Carbohydrates
- Protein

SATURATED FAT

For years, we've been told that too much saturated fat—the kind of fat found in animal foods such as meat and dairy—is bad for us. Food manufacturers take advantage of this belief to push products that are low in fat or have no fat at all. But I'm going to just come out and say it—I believe all the warnings about the dangers of moderate saturated fat intake are either incorrect or, at the very least, exaggerated. A lot of great recent research shows that moderate amounts of saturated fats aren't bad for you. After years of being bombarded with the anti-fat message, this may come as a shock to you. You may be wondering how a staple of medical and dietary advice could be wrong. What's the evidence? To understand that, we need to go back to the origins of the belief that saturated fat is harmful to your health.

SATURATED FATS AND HEART DISEASE

A researcher named Ancel Keys first linked the intake of saturated fats to heart disease back in the 1950s. His influential work was the basis for much of the research and dietary recommendations that followed. Keys examined data from 22 different countries, looking for the relationship between the amount of saturated fat in the diet and the rate of heart disease. He found what he was looking for, but only because he didn't include all of the countries in his final analysis. Instead, he chose seven countries that he felt were most representative. Even though his methods of analysis were groundbreaking for the 1950s, leaving out 15 countries that didn't fit the theory diminished the validity of the results. One of the excluded countries was France. For decades, this led to what was known as the "French paradox." People in France had a lower incidence of heart disease than people in many other countries, despite their high intake of cheese, cream, and other saturated fats.

This anomaly shifted the focus of the investigation as researchers tried to establish what other factors could account for the paradox. In other words, what was countering the negative effects of saturated fat? Rather than look at what the evidence suggested—that saturated fat couldn't be the sole cause of heart disease in other countries—this approach went on to cloud the issue for decades to come.

Based on Ancel Keys' work, a diet high in saturated fat was assumed to be a definite contributing factor to ill health. If a population that ate a lot of saturated fat wasn't getting diseases from it, then some other protective factor must be present. A lot of work went into trying to identify what other factors kept the French from dying of heart disease at high rates. No one seemed to consider that maybe the French paradox wasn't a paradox at all. Maybe it was simply evidence that the assumption about saturated fat was wrong all along. Nevertheless, Keys' conclusions, supported by other similarly flawed population studies in the decades that followed, eventually led to the wholesale acceptance that saturated fats were bad. The entire food industry and culture of health changed accordingly.

Fast forward to today. This nutritional "fact" is finally being actively challenged, even in the mainstream. In 2012, the prestigious and very influential *American Journal of Clinical Nutrition* published a meta-analysis of studies on the dangers of saturated fat. A meta-analysis is essentially a study of numerous studies conducted on one topic. What the authors did was pool together 21 high-quality studies on saturated fat and analyze the combined data. This was no easy task; it included the analysis of nearly 350,000 people who were followed for between 5 and 23 years. The result of this large and widely publicized meta-analysis was that the people who consumed the most saturated fat did *not* have a higher risk of heart disease or stroke.

This was by no means the first study to come to this conclusion. Numerous other studies, including the famous Nurses' Health Study from Harvard, have found no link between the intake of saturated fat and heart disease and stroke. In addition, I am not aware of a single prospective (forward-looking) study that proves the link between higher incidence of heart disease and saturated fat for the general population. A prospective study follows people from when they enter the study forward and measures the outcome based on live data, unlike retrospective studies, which look backward to see what people's recollection of their past habits were.

Of course, multiple studies do show a link between saturated fat and disease, but their validity is questionable. First, the studies don't account for the fact that there might have been something else aside from saturated fat in the diet that contributed to disease. Ancel Keys, for instance, didn't take smoking and alcohol use into account. In the studies linking saturated fat to heart disease, for example, it appears that those who ate more saturated fat also ate more sugar—and, as I'll explain later, sugar is the real villain. In some of the studies, subjects also ate more trans fat, a highly processed form of fat made from vegetable oils that is definitely related to an increased risk of disease. When we look at food intake, we need to look at the bigger picture to establish patterns. Studying one dietary component in isolation is very difficult.

In addition, the methods used for many of the saturated fat studies are subject to inaccuracies. For instance, one method is to have subjects recall what they ate over the last 24 hours; that information is then used as the basis of the study. This approach is frequently used because it's easy to measure, but what someone ate in the last 24 hours is not necessarily reflective of that person's overall dietary pattern over many years. Plus, this method relies on people telling the truth or remembering accurately what they actually ate. If you try to remember everything you ate over the past 24 hours, you would almost certainly forget something; you would also have trouble providing accurate information about your portion sizes. The dietary recall approach goes some way toward explaining why no prospective studies about the health effects of saturated fat have come to the same conclusions as the retrospective studies.

Publication bias also plays a role in how saturated fat studies are interpreted and how their conclusions enter mainstream medicine. Medical journals are flooded with many more articles than they have room to publish. A small group at the journal must choose what is included and what is rejected. Studies that support the prevailing assumptions are far more likely to be published than contradictory studies. Current beliefs aren't always challenged. The authors of the meta-analysis I mentioned above put it this way: "Studies with significant associations tended to be received more favorably for publication." In other words, studies were more likely to be rejected if their conclusions went against the prevailing view on saturated fat.

THE CHOLESTEROL LINK

What about studies that show that saturated fat raises your level of low-density lipoproteins, better known as LDL or bad cholesterol? This probably matters a lot less than what the health establishment has been telling you for decades. Cholesterol has been demonized, but your body actually needs it for a wide range of vital functions, including making your cell membranes; manufacturing the hormones aldosterone, cortisol, testosterone, estrogen, and progesterone; and producing vitamin D in your body.

Almost all the cholesterol in your body is manufactured in your liver—you don't absorb much cholesterol from your food. To transport waxy cholesterol through your watery bloodstream, your liver wraps it up in protein to create a lipoprotein. The cholesterol in your body exists in two basic forms: low-density lipoprotein, or LDL cholesterol, and high-density lipoprotein, or HDL cholesterol. You will often see LDL cholesterol referred to as the bad cholesterol and HDL cholesterol as the good cholesterol. That's because LDL cholesterol carries cholesterol from your liver to your cells, where it is taken up as needed. HDL cholesterol carries the unused cholesterol back to your liver, where about half of it gets recycled to make more LDL cholesterol; some is used to make bile acids, and some is recycled for other uses.

Not all LDL is created equal. Some of your LDL particles take the form of pattern B—small, dense particles that are more likely to enter the wall of a blood vessel and cause an atherosclerotic plaque that can lead to a heart attack. Pattern A LDL is characterized by larger, fluffier particles that are less likely to enter the blood vessel wall. Guess which type is predominately elevated by saturated fat? Contrary to what you might think, it's large, fluffy pattern A LDL, which is less likely to stiffen and clog a blood vessel. Guess which type is predominately increased by sugars? You guessed it— the small, dense pattern B LDL that enters blood vessel walls and causes hardening of the arteries.

Like saturated fat, cholesterol has a bad reputation for causing heart disease. But does it? Cholesterol may end up being a bystander to the overall health debate. About half of all people who have heart attacks have a normal cholesterol level—about the same odds as a coin flip. Many medications can lower LDL cholesterol, but with the possible exception of the statin class, these medications have *not* been proven to reduce the risk of heart attack and stroke. For the statin drugs, the only thing we know for sure is that they help prevent second heart attacks in men who have already had one.

Something else is involved. If it were just about the cholesterol, then all medications that lower cholesterol, not just statin drugs, would also reduce the risk of heart attack and stroke. They don't.

I believe that the "something else" is the "stickiness" of the blood vessel wall. You can have a lot of cholesterol particles floating by as your blood circulates, but not much of it sticks. But some people have only a little floating by, yet a lot of it sticks. Why? If you use your insulin efficiently, you have less "stickiness." If you become insulin resistant, the cascade of health effects it causes makes the delicate lining of your blood vessels (the endothelium) much easier to damage—it becomes roughened. Dense LDL particles get stuck in the cracks and rough spots. Think of your cholesterol as metal shavings and your blood vessel wall as an electromagnet. Current treatment for cholesterol is akin to lowering the amount of metal shavings. But wouldn't it be better to just turn off the magnet? That's what improving your insulin efficiency can do for you. And that's what the methodologies in this book, the YOU+ app, and the website will accomplish.

LOW-FAT DIETS

We can't discuss dietary fats without discussing the validity of a low-fat diet for preventing heart disease and stroke. Low-fat diets got a huge boost in the 1990s based on the work of a pioneering cardiologist, Dr. Dean Ornish. His idea was that coronary artery disease could be not only prevented but reversed based on dietary interventions, including a diet that had very little fat. In 1990, he published a study in the influential medical journal *The Lancet* that looked at 20 patients with severe coronary artery disease. After following the Ornish program for a year, and without taking any drugs, the patients showed modest reductions in their degree of blocked arteries. This study represented an important turning point in the medical establishment's perspective. A low-fat diet was now the way to go for preventing heart disease. We have to remember, however, that not only did the patients follow a low-fat vegetarian diet, but they also stopped smoking, did moderate exercise, and attended stress management classes. And of the 28 patients who started the study, only 20 managed to stick with the very restrictive diet. We can't really say how much of the benefit to the patients came from the diet and what came from all the other factors.

Ornish recommended that less than 10 percent of your daily calories should come from fat. This very low-fat approach was also a way to achieve weight loss. His study group participants did lose a lot of weight. Dr. Ornish believed that they lost weight because gram for gram, fat has more calories (9 per gram) than carbohydrates or protein (4 per gram). If you replace fat with protein or carbohydrate, you get fewer calories for the same weight of food. The math may work, but a very low-fat diet is a difficult diet to stick with. Most of us like the feel and taste of fats in food and find them quite satisfying. Thankfully, there's a far easier method to follow, as you'll soon discover.

Ornish was rightly criticized for the size of his study groups—a lot of participants in his programs dropped out. Also, the participants were all white males. Even so, the supposed connection Dr. Ornish made between diet and coronary heart disease was groundbreaking. But, just as with the other saturated fat studies we have discussed, what probably played an even more important role was what else was cut out of the diet. Dr. Ornish's patients ate very little refined or added sugars. I believe that it's the lack of sugar, not the lack of fat, that helped his patients.

I don't know about you, but when I look at things like the French paradox, the fact that about half of all people who have heart attacks have normal cholesterol levels, and recent research showing that other diets are superior to low-fat diets in preventing disease, my "common sense meter" is activated. There must be something else involved other than the usual suspects of saturated fats and high LDL cholesterol. If you also consider the data on people in the modern era who eat a diet that is very low in carbohydrates and high in saturated fat (the Inuit people of the Arctic region, for instance), you see that they don't seem to have higher rates of heart disease. In fact, their rates are lower. While I don't recommend a very low carbohydrate, very high saturated fat approach, the evidence in favor of fewer carbs and more fat is strong enough that we clearly need to think differently about saturated fat and cholesterol.

The main change in thinking about saturated fat is that it's not harmful in moderate amounts. That doesn't mean a free license to eat it with reckless abandon. Excess weight, no matter how you gain it, leads to insulin resistance and high blood insulin levels—underlying forces we must reckon with. There's also evidence that too much fat intake can alter the composition of our intestinal bacteria (we'll discuss that more in the next chapter), and this can also affect our weight. What the new understanding about saturated fats does mean, however, is that we can eat more of it than previously thought. That makes healthy eating a lot more doable because your food will be more enjoyable and satisfying.

DAIRY FOODS

What does the revelation about saturated fat mean for dairy products in your diet? Given what we now know about saturated fat, do we really have to stick with low-fat dairy all the time? Again, the subject has been extensively studied. One study by Harvard researchers published in 2010 in the *Annals of Internal Medicine* tracked levels of dairy fat consumption by the measurement of something called trans-palmitoleic acid in the blood of nearly 4,000 study participants. Because trans-palmitoleic acid is a marker of dairy fat consumption, the more dairy fat in your diet, the more of this substance is found in your blood. What researchers found is that participants with higher levels of trans-palmitoleic acid were healthier than those with lower levels. They had less body fat, higher good cholesterol levels, lower triglycerides, smaller waist circumferences, and importantly, less insulin resistance.

Another study published in 2002 in the *Journal of the American Medical Association* found that increased dairy consumption protected overweight individuals from getting heavier and developing insulin resistance. A comparison of the highest to the lowest dairy consumers revealed that the highest were 72 percent less likely to develop metabolic syndrome and that each unit increase of daily consumption lowered the risk by 21 percent. Those are pretty impressive results. Other studies have shown that some of this may be due to how dairy affects the response of gastrointestinal hormones.

What kind of dairy you consume may make a difference. Studies have shown that fermented dairy, such as cheese and yogurt, may be the best forms of dairy. Unfortunately, ice cream did not fare well in these comparisons of various dairy types.

It isn't yet clear why dairy products are so protective, but there are many theories. Two dairy components that seem to have a lot of merit are whey protein and something called conjugated linoleic acid (CLA). Whey protein can be very valuable as part of your nutrient timing strategy—so valuable that I'll be discussing it more in Chapter 12. CLA has been linked to lower rates of heart disease and cancer, less body fat, and decreased insulin resistance. The fat in dairy foods contains significant amounts of CLA, which has set off a gold rush for CLA supplements. But before you join in, bear in mind that CLA is naturally found in two slightly different forms in dairy food; together, they occur in a 9:1 ratio. The ratio in supplements is usually 1:1. In fact, some researchers believe that manufactured CLA, which is far from its natural form, may actually have the opposite effect and increases insulin resistance. Stay away from this supplement. As I'll discuss more in Chapter 5, stick to dairy products instead.

Although we benefit from dairy, again, this isn't a free license for unlimited consumption of it. You can't put cheese on everything, and you need to watch out for added sugar in dairy foods such as yogurt. With that in mind, incorporate more dairy into your diet plan to make it better and more enjoyable. Personally, in our home, we have switched from skim milk to 2 percent milk. If I want a snack, I may reach for a piece of natural cheese (not processed cheese or "cheese food"), and I don't hesitate to put a little real cream in my coffee.

RED MEAT

Largely a casualty of the anti-saturated fat dogma, for decades, red meat was considered guilty until proven innocent. I believe that we shouldn't eat huge amounts of red meat, but for reasons other than its saturated fat content. The high iron levels in red meat, as well as how a substance called carnitine is broken down in your digestion, may be problematic. How the meat is prepared may also have health impacts. In spite of all that, red meat certainly can have a place in our diet plan.

Like the studies on saturated fats, the studies conducted on the effects of red meat consumption were often grouped with other nutritional issues or negative behaviors. For example, in studies that looked at the prevalence of a disease across large groups, the people who ate a lot of red meat were found to have more health problems. But was it the red meat that caused them, or was it because the red meat eaters were often heavier to start with and ate fewer fruits and vegetables? In many of these studies, the meat eaters were also less likely to exercise or more likely to be smokers.

What many of the studies seemed to show was that while smokers, for instance, also tend to eat more meat, it is impossible to say that their health issues were a result of their diet.

Unless the consumption of red meat is the only variable among the test subjects, we can't draw any conclusions about it. Doing so, as many studies have, is just bad science. We already know, for example, that being heavier is a risk factor for cancer. How would we know whether the findings of a study showing a link between obesity and cancer risk were because the subjects were heavier from eating more red meat or because of some other dietary or behavioral component?

Perhaps the biggest problem when trying to establish the truth about red meat is that until recently, the studies on meat intake combined the consumption of processed meats with fresh meat. Processed meats, such as bologna, hot dogs, bacon, ham, and sausage, are full of preservatives, colorings, flavorings, and other unnatural additions, plus a lot of added salt. Some meats are smoked, which is also known to be problematic.

A large meta-analysis of 20 studies that was published on this subject in 2010 separated out processed from unprocessed meats for the first time. The combined studies involved around one million people. Unprocessed red meat turned out not to be a risk factor for heart disease or diabetes. Processed meat, on the other hand, was a risk factor for both. Disturbingly, the equivalent of only one hot dog a day increased the risk for coronary heart disease by a staggering 42 percent. Another study, published in 2011 in the *American Journal of Clinical Nutrition*, found that processed, but not unprocessed, red meat was associated with a higher risk of stroke.

More research also needs to be done to compare different methods of feeding animals and the resultant health effects of the meat produced. For instance, grass-fed beef has higher levels of the protective CLA we discussed earlier in the section on dairy.

Given all of the recent evidence, I believe that eating unprocessed red meat in moderation does have a place in a healthy diet, particularly when used as part of a strategy to keep weight at an optimal level. However, we *should* significantly limit our intake of processed meat—the health data about its bad effects are concerning. That's not to say I'm never going to have the occasional serving of bacon, because I will. I don't do it regularly, just as an occasional indulgence.

POLYUNSATURATED FATS

The saturated fat I discussed above comes primarily from animal foods, such as butter and meat. Saturated fats are usually solid at room temperature—butter is a good example. Polyunsaturated fats are chemically a little different from saturated fats; some of their hydrogen molecules are replaced by an extra bond with carbon. That makes polyunsaturated fats liquid at room temperature. Polyunsaturated fats include corn oil, safflower seed oil, sunflower seed oil, flaxseed oil, and, most important, fish oil.

Polyunsaturated fats fall into two very distinct categories:

- Omega-3 fatty acids
- Omega-6 fatty acids

Your body needs both kinds of fat—the omega in the names is a chemical term for the structure of one end of the fat molecule. The omega-3 and -6 fatty acids are what nutritionists call "essential," meaning that our bodies can't make them, so we have to get them from our food. Although both types are necessary, they behave very differently in the body. As it turns out, what's really important is the amount of each that our body gets over and above our baseline requirement. For good health, we need to have a good balance of each fat—the ratio between the two is important.

Omega-6 fatty acids are predominately found in vegetable oils, particularly corn oil, safflower oil, and sunflower oil. One of their major functions in the body is to form breakdown chemicals, which increase inflammation. An excess of breakdown chemicals is associated with many chronic diseases, including heart disease, cancer, Alzheimer's disease, arthritis, and depression.

Omega-3 fatty acids are mainly found in seafood (particularly oily fish), nuts, seeds, whole grains, beans, and green leafy vegetables. Their major function in the body is the opposite of omega-6 fatty acids. Omega-3s increase the formation of chemicals used for repair and are anti-inflammatory.

OMEGA-6 TO OMEGA-3 RATIO

Although the Western diet has changed dramatically in the last century, for much of human history, the intake ratio of omega-6 to omega-3 fatty acids was probably in the neighborhood of 2.5:1. In other words, we ate 2.5 times more omega-6 fatty acids than omega-3 fatty acids. Starting in the early 20th century, however, processed foods became a much bigger part of our diet. Refined vegetable oils became more prevalent in our diet, which increased our intake of omega-6s. At the same time, our intake of omega-3 foods declined. As a consequence of these changes, the ratio of omega-6 to omega-3 fatty acids in the typical American diet has increased dramatically, to around 16:1 (some experts think it is even higher). I believe this distorted and unbalanced ratio has contributed to the overall decline of health and well-being in this country from the pro-inflammatory effects of excess omega-6 fatty acids.

Some researchers argue that since these fatty acids are essential, excess amounts of them are unlikely to harm us. They point out that the production of the most inflammatory chemicals is tightly regulated by the body. Significant evidence to the contrary, however, says that our unbalanced ratio of fatty acids is indeed very harmful. Reducing the amount of omega-6 fatty acids and increasing the amount of omega-3s to get a better ratio has been shown to be effective. Recent study findings include:

- Reduction of the ratio to 5:1 had a beneficial effect on asthma, while a ratio of 10:1 increased asthma symptoms.

- Reduction of the ratio to 4:1 reduced total mortality by 70 percent in the secondary prevention of heart disease.

- Reduction of the ratio to 3:1 reduced the symptoms of rheumatoid arthritis.

- Reduction of the ratio to 2.5:1 reduced cancer cell proliferation in colorectal cancer.

This radical shift in our fatty acid intake means that we are now heavily tilted against the prevailing dietary pattern of generations of our ancestors. We can, however, affect this ratio in two ways. We can decrease our intake of omega-6, since most people get more than enough to meet the essential requirements, and we can increase our intake of omega-3.

We can increase our omega-3 levels by eating more foods that contain it, particularly fish, nuts, and whole grains. We can also take supplements of fish oil. To cut down on the omega-6 fatty acids in our diet, we can reduce the amount of junk and processed foods in our diet. These foods, such as store-bought cookies, crackers, and chips, are made with cheap vegetable oils that are high in omega-6 fatty acids. We can also decrease our omega-6 intake simply by changing the oils we use to cook our food. This is easy to do: simply swap polyunsaturated fats, especially vegetable oils such as corn oil, for monounsaturated fats like olive oil.

MONOUNSATURATED FATS

All edible oils have more than one type of fat in them, but they're categorized by their main component. Monounsaturated fats are missing just one hydrogen atom, which is replaced by an extra bond to just one carbon atom—that's where the mono-part, meaning one, comes from. Olive oil, canola oil, peanut oil, and the oils found in nuts, seeds, and avocados are all primarily monounsaturated fats. By using these fats for cooking, you get benefits beyond just reducing your intake of omega-6. These fats have been shown to have a beneficial effect on cholesterol, blood pressure, and inflammation, and may reduce the risk of cancer.

It is also important to understand what happens to cooking oil when it is heated. Polyunsaturated oils, particularly when heated for a long time or when frequently reheated (as they are in deep fryers), form a compound known as HNE that has been linked to cancer and heart disease, among other ailments. Although some non-monounsaturated fats, such as butter, don't produce this toxic compound when heated, using a monounsaturated fat like olive oil, which also doesn't produce HNE, is a healthier and safer option than polyunsaturated oils. Another oil to consider for high-temperature cooking is coconut oil because it is very stable in this regard. Even though coconut oil has a high saturated fat content, it has not shown any adverse health effects. In any event, use cooking oil only once and keep it below its smoke point (that helps avoid kitchen fires, too).

MEDITERRANEAN DIET

The people of the Mediterranean region use a lot of monoun-saturated oil in their diet. This dietary approach is characterized by the use of olive oil as the main fat; dietary fat also comes from fish (an excellent source of omega-3 fats), poultry, whole grains, fruits, vegetables, nuts, dairy products, and limited (just once or twice a week) consumption of red meat. The diet contains very little added sugar. Overall, people who eat the typical Mediter-ranean diet get about 40 percent of their calories from fat. In general, in Mediterranean countries like Greece and Italy, the focus is on enjoying the flavor of good, fresh food while spend-ing more time eating and sharing the experience with others. Moderate consumption of red wine is also an important aspect.

The Mediterranean approach to diet has long been known to keep people healthy and long-lived. Since the 1960s, the diet has been carefully studied to learn exactly how beneficial it is. To cite just one good example, a study published in the *Archives of Internal Medicine* followed the diets of 380,000-plus men and women over ten years. Those who ate a Mediterranean-style diet reduced their risk of death by 20 percent over the ten years com-pared to the participants who ate a more American-style diet. In other studies that compared the Mediterranean diet directly to a low-fat diet, the Mediterranean diet was found to be much better at preventing heart disease.

The Mediterranean diet is the basis for the Dietary Approaches to Stop Hypertension (DASH) diet, now widely recommended by doctors for people with heart disease. The value of the DASH diet was shown in the famed Lyons Heart Diet Study, published in the prestigious journal *Circulation* in 2001. Participants in the study had all already had a heart attack. They were divided into two groups, one to eat the normal Western-style diet (high in sugar and refined carbohydrates and low in good fats) and one to eat a Mediterranean-style diet. The researchers wanted to know which diet would do more to reduce the risk of worsening heart disease over five years. They quickly discovered that the Mediterranean diet was much more effective—mortality from all causes in the Mediterranean group was reduced 70 percent. The group randomized to the Mediterranean-type diet had 14 cardiac events, compared with 44 in the group randomized to the Western diet. The results were so compelling that the study was ended a year early.

Most important, in all the studies, the people following the Mediterranean diet were *not* asked to reduce their calories. They ate well, felt satisfied by their food, and improved their health. This approach is very close to what we are looking for. When my patients tell me they follow it, I don't object at all. I do, however, believe that certain aspects of the diet can be further improved for even greater benefit. In particular, the Mediterranean diet is fairly high in carbohydrates from bread, pasta, rice, and other starchy foods. It's not as high in protein as desired for creating the optimal GI hormone response. And if you follow the official DASH diet, you don't get much added fat—dipping your food in olive oil, for instance, isn't part of the plan. People who are overweight and follow a Mediterranean-style diet do better and lose weight more easily if they cut back on carbohydrates and increase their protein intake. And because carbohydrate foods make us produce insulin to metabolize the glucose they contain, they make us produce insulin that we may not use efficiently.

CARBOHYDRATES

Although you've probably heard references to "good carbs" and "bad carbs," these simplistic monikers don't really tell the full story. In fact, these terms may even be misleading.

Carbohydrates are sugary or starchy foods that break down quickly into glucose when they're digested. Some carbohydrates break down faster than others. Generally speaking, the more refined or processed a carbohydrate food is, the faster its glucose will hit your bloodstream and the more rapidly you will need to produce insulin to handle it. For example, brown rice, which is less processed, breaks down more slowly than white rice. While it's true that less processed is desirable, does this make white rice a bad carb? Not in the context of a healthy diet. Think about it. People in Asian cultures enjoy very good health and longevity while eating lots of white rice. And there are European cultures that enjoy good health and longevity in spite of eating lots of potatoes, bread, and pasta. Understanding carbohydrates and their role in our diet is clearly not as black and white as good versus bad.

NATURAL VERSUS ADDED SUGARS

Your body's primary source of energy is glucose, a type of sugar. Glucose is our energy currency, our principle source of fuel. Glucose is found naturally in almost everything we eat that has an element of sweetness or starchiness. It's found in fruits and vegetables, grains, rice, potatoes, pasta, and bread, among others. Our bodies are capable of handling this sugar and can normally do so very efficiently.

Problems occur, however, when you ask your body to metabolize forms of sugar besides glucose. The common sugar we use ourselves is sucrose, or ordinary white table sugar. Sucrose is actually two molecules linked together: one glucose molecule and one fructose molecule. The addition of fructose makes sucrose taste a little sweeter than glucose.

We add sucrose to lots of foods, from sugar in our coffee to sweet baked goods—and also to many processed foods that don't even taste sweet, like creamy canned soups and salad dressings. But the most commonly added form of sugar is something called high-fructose corn syrup (HFCS), which is used extensively in all kinds of processed foods and beverages. HFCS gets a lot of bad press—deservedly so, in my opinion. Because we eat a lot of processed foods and beverages, we consume much more HFCS than table sugar. Sucrose and high-fructose corn syrup are actually extremely similar. Remember how sucrose is one glucose and one fructose molecule put together for a 50–50 ratio? Well, HFCS is generally 55 percent fructose and 45 percent glucose, so the amount of fructose isn't much greater. In both table sugar and high-fructose corn syrup, it's the fructose that's the problem. It doesn't really matter if the fructose from added sugar is 50 percent from table sugar or 55 percent from HFCS. It's bad for your health. The reason is that fructose is metabolized by your body very differently from glucose.

This was first suggested back in the early 20th century by Frederick Banting, the researcher who won the Nobel Prize for his discovery of insulin. The start of the 1900s was the first period in human history to experience a large spike in added sugar consumption. In fact, sugar consumption doubled in America between 1890 and 1920 as sugar become cheaper and more widely available. Banting suggested that sugar consumption was the cause of the 15-fold rise in deaths from type 2 diabetes in New York City compared with the 1860s. As always, there was a counterargument. Other researchers suggested that because type 2 diabetes was rare in other cultures such as Japan, and people in those cultures ate a lot of rice, and rice is a carbohydrate, and a carbohydrate is a form of sugar, it must not be the added sugars that were causing the spike in diabetes deaths. It was a convenient albeit tenuous argument, and despite knowledge to the contrary, it is still around today.

To make matters even worse, there has been another spike in added sugar consumption since the 1980s. There are multiple causes for this, but perhaps the most obvious is the rise in consumption of sugary drinks such as soda, fruit juice, and sports drinks. When high-fructose corn syrup began to be used to make these drinks, their price went down and consumption soared. It's no accident that the rapid rise in obesity paralleled the rise in sugar consumption that began during this time. Today, the increase in the rate of sugar consumption is flattening, but it is still at much, much higher levels than decades ago. Until we get our sugar intake back down to where it was before that explosive increase, our country's weight problem will be extremely difficult to manage.

The less obvious culprit in this problem is the push to lower the amount of fat in our diet that started in the 1990s from American health authorities. While this effort has been successful, with the percentage of calories from fat falling from about 40 percent to 30 percent, it had an unintended side effect. To cut the fat in processed foods, the manufacturers used added sugar instead. They had to. Low-fat processed foods taste lousy unless sugar, in the form of sucrose or high-fructose corn syrup, is added to make up for the missing flavor and texture from fat. The addition of sugar also helped with the browning of cooked foods. It decreased cooking time and increased shelf life. That was great for the food manufacturers, but not so great for consumers. They ended up eating even more, because low-fat foods aren't as satisfying. Instead of eating a few full-fat cookies, they ended up eating a lot of low-fat cookies.

The increased sugar (sucrose) and HFCS consumption meant people were eating both more glucose and more fructose. That's where the key difference between glucose and fructose comes in. When sucrose is broken down in your digestive system, the glucose can be used quickly by every cell in your body for energy. The fructose, however, has to be metabolized by your liver before it can be used for fuel. So, when you eat a food that has a lot of sucrose in it, less glucose than fructose gets to your liver to be metabolized, because it's being used elsewhere first. This means that your liver must process about three times the volume of carbohydrate when faced with table sugar (with its additional fructose content) compared with glucose. About 20 percent of the glucose you eat reaches your liver, whereas almost 60 percent of the added sugar you eat, including the fructose, reaches your liver.

The increased volume is only part of the problem. Once they reach your liver, fructose and glucose are metabolized differently. Fructose is much more likely to end up being stored as fat in the liver. That is a huge difference with obvious ramifications. A liver full of fat results in many health consequences, including an increase in insulin resistance and its resultant higher insulin levels in the blood.

This is a good time to bring up alcohol consumption, as alcohol is metabolized by the liver in much the same way as fructose. Because of this, people who regularly drink alcohol tend to store a lot of fat in the liver. Insulin resistance can follow, for all of the same reasons. I know there are many studies showing that moderate alcohol consumption can be beneficial. If you are carrying more weight than you should, however, the tables may turn on you.

How your body reacts to the different sugars also affects your appetite hormones. When you eat foods high in glucose, you affect your leptin level. Your fat cells release leptin, which essentially tells your brain that you're full and don't need to eat. Glucose also suppresses the hunger hormone ghrelin, which tells us we're hungry. Fructose, however, doesn't turn on the leptin signal that you're full or turn off the ghrelin signal that you're hungry to the same degree. That's bad news for your waistline. Add to this the effect that high insulin levels have on blocking the effect of leptin in the brain, and you have a recipe for disaster.

FRUCTOSE AND INTESTINAL DAMAGE

Increased gut permeability is an additional problem that can be caused by excess fructose in the diet. Ordinarily, the cells that line your intestines fit very tightly together. The spaces between them, known as junctions, open to allow molecules of digested food to pass from your intestines into your bloodstream. When the tight junctions are working properly, only tiny particles of nutrients pass through; bacteria, toxins, undigested food, and larger particles are kept safely within the intestines. But if your gut bacteria are out of balance or if you have a diet high in processed foods full of fructose (the two often go hand in hand), the intestines can become more permeable—the junctions are no longer as tight as they should be. Larger particles and toxins from gut bacteria can then pass through the junctions and enter your bloodstream. In severe cases, you develop leaky gut syndrome, which has a range of unpleasant symptoms, including abdominal pain, bloating, diarrhea, and poor immunity. More commonly, increased intestinal permeability is less severe but just as damaging. The toxins entering your bloodstream cause mild overall inflammation, which in turn shifts the balance of your body's repair and breakdown chemicals toward breakdown. You might not even realize you have a problem, but we now have a lot of good evidence showing that ongoing low-level inflammation may well be a root cause of obesity and insulin resistance, as well as heart disease.

How can you fix intestinal permeability? Reducing or removing high-fructose processed foods from your diet is crucial. Take probiotic supplements to help restore a better balance of beneficial bacteria in your gut. Use the amino acid supplement glutamine to help heal the damaged intestinal wall. The improvement will probably happen gradually, over a period of several weeks. To help keep intestinal permeability from coming back, continue with glutamine on a daily basis. I'll explain more about the value of probiotics for everyone in Chapter 5. I'll explain more about glutamine when we get to Chapter 12.

A couple of years ago, one of my patients really showed me how intestinal permeability can cause stubborn weight gain. Becky, a woman in her 30s, felt bloated all the time and was having trouble losing weight even though she had improved her diet quite a bit by cutting out most processed foods. I thought the problem might be lingering intestinal permeability from her previous poor diet. Becky started taking 5 grams of glutamine daily. Her bloating soon improved. She also felt better, was more energetic, and was finally able to break through a plateau in her weight.

FRUCTOSE THE NATURAL WAY

What about the fructose that occurs naturally in our foods? It's found in fruit, as the name suggests, and also in some vegetables. The difference is that naturally occurring fructose is packaged with lots of fiber. That makes us feel full long before we can eat too much of it; also, the fiber slows down your absorption of the fructose.

A fruit such as an apple is rich in both fructose and fiber—they give the apple both its sweetness and its crunch. Even sugar cane has so much fiber in it that it's almost like a piece of wood. The cane has to be crushed and heavily processed to extract the sugar.

Due to the natural fiber in fruits and vegetables, it's hard to consume more than 35 grams of fructose each day. An apple has about 13 grams of fructose and about 5 grams of fiber. You would have a hard time eating three apples in a row, but it would be easy to eat three chocolate chip cookies in a row! The cookies have all the fructose but none of the fiber. By comparison, a 20-ounce soda has about 36 grams of fructose. Many people drink down several large sodas in the course of a day.

On the other hand, the naturally occurring glucose in our foods is broken down in a desirable and efficient way—assuming, of course, that it has no added sugar and hasn't been overly processed and stripped of fiber and nutrients. Glucose from foods like rice, pasta, potatoes, and whole-grain bread will be metabolized first by the body, and then stored less by the liver. Among historically healthy European and Asian cultures, high-quality carbohydrates are part of a healthy lifestyle. Consider the potato. The whole potato with its skin is very different than the french fry. The whole potato provides glucose and fiber to the body; the french fry has had all of its fiber removed and is then fried in reused polyunsaturated oil. In the same way, whole-grain bread is higher in fiber and nutrients than white bread. The key difference is processing—the less of it, the better.

GLYCEMIC INDEX (GI)

In a nutshell, the glycemic index (GI) describes how quickly 100 grams of a carbohydrate-containing food such as sugar or white bread will make your blood sugar rise. It's a trendy term that's now often used when talking about good and bad carbohydrates. The GI was developed to be a useful basic concept that would help people with diabetes understand what foods are best for them to eat. However, the GI is also misleading for several reasons. For a start, as you now know, not all carbohydrates are created equal. As it turns out, fructose actually has a very low glycemic index, but this doesn't make it desirable. In addition, the glycemic index is measured when a food is eaten in isolation, but few foods are genuinely eaten only by themselves. In reality, we almost always combine several foods when we eat. It's almost impossible to calculate the glycemic index even of something as simple as a peanut butter and jelly sandwich, even though we know the numbers for the individual components. Another important shortcoming of GI is it doesn't take into account how much of a food is eaten.

The glycemic index has so many drawbacks that it's not that helpful. A related concept, the glycemic load, is much more useful. The glycemic load looks at the total effect of an entire meal, both in terms of the type of carbohydrate eaten and the amount consumed. The amounts used in calculating the glycemic load can be calculated for any portion size, not just the standardized 100-gram amount used to calculate the glycemic index of a food. By combining foods in the right proportions, we can optimize glycemic load to our advantage.

SUGAR INTAKE STUDIES

Much of the research on the dangers of added sugars has centered on the most easily studied form of intake: sugary drinks like soda, fruit juices with added sugars, and sports drinks. A 2010 study from the Harvard School of Public Health is one that I believe typifies what is going on in this area. It was a meta-analysis (a study of studies) of 11 high-quality studies that included over 310,000 participants. In their meta-analysis, the researchers found that drinking at least one sugar-laden drink every day increased the risk of developing the full-blown metabolic syndrome by 20 percent, compared to people who didn't drink any. When it came to type 2 diabetes, people who drank the most sugary drinks had a 26 percent greater risk of developing the metabolic syndrome than those who didn't drink any.

The authors of the study pointed out that this effect was in some ways independent of the significant weight gain also seen in the subjects. In other words, the higher incidence of insulin resistance among the sugary drink consumers was possibly due to the fructose content in these drinks, not just the weight gain they experienced from the increased calories.

Interestingly, this increase of insulin resistance didn't occur when subjects consumed freshly prepared fruit juice with no added sugar. In a separate study in 2010 published in the *Journal of the American College of Nutrition*, researchers found that consumers of no-sugar-added juices had the opposite effect. Those people were leaner, had smaller waists, used insulin more efficiently, and were less likely to have the metabolic syndrome. This would seem to support the conclusions of the Harvard study that the added fructose in soda and other sweetened beverages was indeed playing a role.

Other studies look at added sugars as a whole, not just in drinks. The findings of these studies are equally alarming. They conclude that added sugars are closely associated with weight gain and other components of the metabolic syndrome, such as lower HDL cholesterol and higher triglycerides. A study published in 2014 in *JAMA Internal Medicine* concluded starkly that adults who get 25 percent of their daily calories from sugar have a risk of death from heart disease that is nearly 2.5 times higher than people who consume less than 10 percent of their calories from sugar.

To strengthen any scientific analysis, we have to show that the converse is also true. In other words, if you remove added sugars from the diet, would these health parameters improve?

As you might have guessed, they do. Added sugars simply do not do you any favors. They should be avoided for more reasons than just their empty calories.

ARTIFICIAL SWEETENERS

If added sugars are expanding our waistlines, then isn't the solution simple? Just use artificial sweeteners that have no calories. Voilà, problem solved. At one point, that seemed like a good idea, but it has turned out to be a dangerously misguided assumption. We now know that artificial sweeteners may cause weight gain, the very thing they are supposed to prevent. Artificial sweeteners are found in a lot of food products, but they're most widely used in soft drinks. That makes it easy for researchers to look at diet soda as a marker of artificial sweetener consumption. The results of some recent studies are revealing:

- One study, involving a large number of people who were followed as part of the renowned Framingham Heart Study, produced benchmark research. This study revealed that compared to individuals who drank less than one can of diet soda per day, those who drank one or more diet sodas every day had a 31 percent *greater* risk of being obese and a 30 percent *greater* risk of adding belly fat. They also had a 25 percent *greater* risk of having high blood sugar or high triglycerides.

- In another investigation, drinking just one can of diet soda per day was found to be associated with a 61 percent increase in the risk of heart attack and stroke. The Texas Health Science Center has produced research demonstrating that the waists of those who drank diet soda grew 70 percent more than those who didn't. For each diet soda consumed on average per day, you are 65 percent more likely to become overweight.

- At the same level of consumption, diet soda also increases the risk of diabetes.

- Another study of nearly 10,000 adults found that just one can of diet soda every day *increased* the risk of the full-blown metabolic syndrome by 34 percent.

In short, too much artificial sweetener, or certainly something about diet soda consumption, is seriously detrimental to your health.

When these findings first began pouring in, the original explanation tried to pin the blame on human behavior. It was felt that it must be something *else* that the diet soda drinkers were doing that was causing the problem, rather than the diet soda itself. This viewpoint reminded me vividly of an event from my childhood.

After my older sister learned to drive, she acquired the ability to bribe her little brother in the rare instance that she needed to. On one such occasion, I had a piece of information that she didn't want anyone to find out about. When I was younger, a quarter would buy my silence, but as I got older I knew I could hold out for more. The eventual price of my silence was to be driven to Dairy Queen for an ice cream treat. It was there that the original diet soda theory was demonstrated. While my sister has always been very fit, she would order a banana split, and for some reason, a Tab (an early diet cola). Early researchers thought that people who ordered diet sodas were simply doing so in greater numbers because they were overindulging elsewhere. In other words, as my sister did, they were making up for indulging in something like a banana split. We now know that there are, in fact, much greater forces at work.

Your taste buds are not the only thing that is fooled by an artificial sweetener. When your body senses that something sweet is coming, it makes the assumption that it's glucose. The gastro-intestinal system prepares for the influx of glucose it believes is coming by switching into storage and processing mode. When the sugar hit never arrives, the body sends out the signal that its needs are not being met, and this may spur further appetite and caloric intake.

The artificial sweeteners may also be fooling our brains. An interesting study used MRI brain scans to compare the brains of people drinking a mixture of water and sugar with others drinking a mixture of water and artificial sweetener that tasted exactly the same. The researchers found the brain's "reward center" responded more completely to sugar than to the artificial sweetener. This means that the brain is more satisfied from a real sweet than a fake one. This has important consequences. When the brain's reward center is unsatisfied, it will keep you craving a sweet fix until it is. You'll keep eating until you satisfy the craving. Unfortunately, repeated exposure also trains your body to prefer sweets. It doesn't take long to get you into a negative cycle of overeating.

WHAT DO WE DO ABOUT CARBOHYDRATES?

The bottom line is that added sugars and artificial sweeteners are bad. We need to significantly restrict them to limit their damage. But what about carbohydrates that naturally break down into glucose? How much of those can we have? Is strict carbohydrate limitation a good idea? Let's find the answers by looking at careful studies that compare low-carb diets to other types of diets.

Low-carbohydrate diets definitely do result in weight loss. A number of good studies suggest that the greatest amount of weight is lost with this method compared to other approaches, such as a low-fat diet. This is probably the biggest advantage of a diet low in carbohydrates and, as such, catches the media's attention. The criticism that low-carb dieting increased the risk of heart disease because you eat more saturated fat instead hasn't held up, as you would have expected from our discussion of fats earlier. The very large and ongoing Nurses' Health Study showed that a diet lower in carbohydrates doesn't result in a higher risk of heart disease, even after 20 years. Again, this is consistent with our analysis of dietary fat. On the contrary, in the Nurses' Health Study, the subjects who ate the most carbohydrates from added sugars and processed foods had nearly double the risk of heart disease as those who ate the least.

Other studies have shown that low-carbohydrate diets have the most beneficial effect on lowering cholesterol and inflammation markers. One study, published in the *New England Journal of Medicine* in 2008, followed subjects for two years and demonstrated that a low-carbohydrate diet was superior to a low-fat diet on lowering these inflammatory parameters. It's also worth noting that a Mediterranean diet had a more beneficial effect on these parameters than a low-fat diet.

The idea behind a low-carbohydrate diet is that less insulin is secreted, resulting in less fat storage. If there isn't enough glucose from carbohydrates to burn, the theory is that the body will turn to its fat reserves for energy, resulting in weight loss. Further weight is often lost in the first days of a low-carbohydrate diet as the body adapts to burning ketoacids, formed when the body breaks down fat for energy. At first, the body tries to flush the ketoacids out by increasing urination. More water is lost at first because your body stores some glucose in your liver and muscles as a substance called glycogen. Every one molecule of glycogen is bound up with four of water, so as you burn down your glycogen stores, you also lose the retained water weight.

Although the quick initial weight loss you might experience on a low-carbohydrate diet is due in part to water loss, that's not why a low-carb diet is superior. One important reason is that while low-carb dieting doesn't require calorie counting or reduction, most people who do it find that they naturally tend to consume fewer calories. The diet is higher in fat and protein, which are more satiating, so low-carb dieters just don't feel as hungry; when they do feel hungry, they are quickly satisfied with smaller portions. Feeling satisfied by fewer calories is important to the YOU+ health goals, so we'll look at this more closely later in this book.

The biggest issue I have with carbohydrate-restricted diets is that they assume that the only reason we eat fewer carbs—or even eat at all—is to manage our weight. Often, a diet low in carbohydrates also restricts fruits and starchy vegetables, which many people find difficult to live with over the long term. Low-carb diets restrict added sugars and usually include increased protein intake, both of which are advantageous, but overall, low-carb diets are seriously lacking in variety and enjoyment.

There's a better way to get a healthy, varied diet that will lead to better insulin efficiency, satisfaction, and weight loss: follow the simple YOU+ ratio of protein to carbohydrates and eat as many fruits and veggies as you want. I'll explain this in detail in Chapter 5. For now, let's look at the role protein plays in your nutrition.

PROTEIN

Diets that are higher in protein do three important things:

1. They often result in the greatest amount of weight loss.

2. You are much more likely to keep the weight off on a higher-protein diet.

3. Higher-protein diets achieve weight loss through greater loss of fatty tissue while also preserving lean tissue.

The reason a higher-protein diet works goes back to one of the foundation concepts we discussed in Chapter 1: the hormones that are produced by the gut and your own body fat. Remember that leptin, ghrelin, and other hormones send signals to tell us whether we've eaten enough or need to eat more. The hormone signals do this in many different ways, from signaling our brain to stop eating to slowing how fast our stomachs empty.

We know from studies that our levels of gut hormones correlate well with our food intake for the next meal, as well as for the rest of the day. In other words, if we can naturally optimize our hormone levels through what we eat, we will want less, eat less, and be less hungry the rest of the day.

Eating a meal with additional protein helps move our gut hormones toward their optimal levels. Remember peptide YY from Chapter 1, the hormone that signals the hypothalamus? After a high-protein meal, levels of this hormone more than double compared to the rise from a normal-protein meal. Eating more protein also increases the level of incretin hormones, which keep your blood sugar levels from rising too high. Because incretin hormones directly affect the insulin system, optimizing them gives you a major advantage in the fight against insulin resistance. A higher-protein meal increases incretin hormones by 20 percent compared to a normal-protein meal.

Something called diet-induced thermogenesis may also be contributing to the higher-protein edge. Diet-induced thermogenesis is a measure of how much a food increases your metabolic rate compared to its calorie content. It's typically expressed as a percentage. Protein has a thermogenesis value of around 25 percent. Fats are around 3 percent, and carbohydrates are around 7 percent. It's easy to see how a higher-protein diet can rev up your metabolism.

People who exercise regularly need more protein than those who don't. The dietary plan in this book, the YOU+ app, and the website takes your personal exercise regimen into account and dovetails it with the dietary recommendations to give you the biggest advantage.

Athletes have long known that they maintain more muscle and lose more fat during weight loss when they eat a higher-protein diet. A number of recent studies confirm this belief. For example, a study done at the University of Illinois revealed that the addition of a higher-protein diet to a regimen of resistance training resulted in better preservation of lean muscle mass and more fat loss during weight loss than other diets. A study from Stanford University published in the *Journal of the American Medical Association* added to these findings by showing that following a higher-protein diet for 12 months resulted in greater loss of fat.

There has even been a study of increased protein intake on blood pressure. The DASH diet I mentioned earlier is similar in many ways to a diet low in saturated fat. Following the DASH diet for just eight weeks has been shown to lower high blood pressure. A recent study in the *Archives of Internal Medicine* showed that stroke and heart attacks were significantly reduced in women who followed the DASH diet over nearly 25 years.

Another research group, however, has shown that by replacing some of the carbohydrates in the DASH diet with protein and monounsaturated fats, even further blood pressure reduction could be accomplished. This raises the possibility that replacing some of the carbohydrates in this same way could lower stroke and heart disease as well.

Although many people still mistakenly believe that a higher-protein diet can damage healthy kidneys, unless there is inherent undetected kidney disease, this just isn't the case.

The related belief that a higher-protein diet weakens the bones is similarly unfounded. That high levels of protein in the diet are perfectly safe is summed up by the U.S. Food and Nutrition Board, the people who bring you the official recommended daily allowances (RDA) of nutritional items. The Board also sets the Tolerable Upper Intake Level (UL) for nutrients. This is the maximum level at which you can ingest something before experiencing some sort of a negative result, such as a vitamin overload. The Board doesn't set a UL for protein, acknowledging that you can't really overdose on it.

Now that you know what you need to about fats, carbohydrates, and proteins, we're almost ready to put that knowledge into action with a diet and exercise plan tailored precisely to your needs. But first, we need to cover a few other topics that are relevant to weight loss and health, including the role of genetics, gut bacteria, and the social aspects of well-being.

CHAPTER 4
CONQUERING HEADWINDS

I N EARLIER CHAPTERS, WE'VE covered what to eat and why in an effort to separate fact from fiction. But before we discuss the YOU+ nutrition plan in more detail, it's important to acknowledge that when it comes to health and well-being, it's not just about what you eat. Other factors can or are assumed to influence results. Three aspects in particular seem to have a major impact on your health:

- Genetics

- Gut bacteria

- Social aspects of weight loss

GENETICS

Ever since the 1980s, when gene sequencing became much easier, the idea that our genes control our health and well-being has become widespread. According to the media, there's a gene that controls everything, including our weight. But are we really controlled by our genes? Not entirely—your genetics are more complex than that. Can we change our inherited characteristics? Can we exert control over how our genes function? Is it possible to make effective decisions about our weight and fitness, even if our genetic inheritance is stacked against us? The answer to all these questions is a resounding "Yes!"

Genes do matter when it comes to our weight and fitness, but they're only part of the story. We know from studies of adoptees and twins raised apart, for example, that genes do control part of our weight. Within our families, however, we share not only genetics but also environment—and environment makes the difference. Our fate is rarely sealed by some genetic lottery. Instead, it's our environment, choices, and actions that in the end help us stay fit and at a healthy weight. We have a saying in medicine that's very true: genes load the gun, but environment pulls the trigger. You can't change your genes, but you can change how your environment makes your genes work.

Sometimes it's hard to distinguish between the genetic and the environmental. Ask yourself this: Is the child of overweight parents overweight himself because of some genetic disposition toward obesity, or is he overweight because of the food he is given in the home and the lifestyle choices he sees his parents make and believes to be normal? It's most likely both. This poor kid is in an environment that favors weight gain, whether or not he also has a genetic tendency toward it. He's being set up for a lifetime of obesity and poor health at an age when he can't do anything about it.

My patient Jim, now in his 30s, is one of four kids. When I first saw him, he weighed in at nearly 300 pounds; his siblings and parents are all equally obese. Growing up, being seriously overweight just seemed normal to Jim. But then Jim had a scare about his heart health, one serious enough to jolt him into changing his ways. We worked together to make substantial changes in his lifestyle. Jim cut out junk food, increased his intake of fruits and veggies, and stopped drinking soda. He added in regular resistance and cardio exercise. Over the course of about a year, Jim lost 80 pounds. He felt great. Since then, Jim has kept off the weight and has kept up his exercise program. He's learned that obesity wasn't his genetic fate—it was his environment that was the problem.

Regardless of whether it's nature or nurture, the simple truth is that you can make the most or the least of the genetics you were born with. If you know you have control over your health despite your genes, then you are much more likely to take responsibility for your own well-being and make healthy choices. You won't just shrug your shoulders and say, "It's genetic."

Do you really have control over your genes? Yes, and to a surprising extent. Today we know a lot more about the epigenome—all the factors that control how a gene is expressed. Just because you have a gene doesn't mean it is going to be expressed (carry out a specific function). External factors can turn a gene on or off. For example, someone might have a gene that predisposes him to lung cancer. But if that person isn't exposed to tobacco smoke, which can turn on the gene, he almost certainly won't develop lung cancer. In this case, his environment and choices alter the outcome of his genetic heritage. The trigger to his loaded lung cancer gun is never pulled.

What about what we do with diet, exercise, and fitness? How do they alter the way our genes speak to our bodies? One study published in 2008 in the *Proceedings of the National Academy of Sciences* was a harbinger of how our thinking would change about our genetics. The study followed 30 men who had been diagnosed with low-risk prostate cancer, meaning they didn't need immediate surgery or other medical intervention. For three months, the men participated in an intensive program where they exercised, ate a lot of fruits, vegetables, and whole grains, and learned to manage their stress. At the end of three months, the men had additional prostate biopsies. Gene activity in these biopsies was compared to the gene activity in the original biopsies that detected the cancer. The researchers found that following three months of favorable lifestyle changes caused alterations in the activity of about 500 genes, including 48 that were turned on and 453 that were turned off. The activity of disease-preventing genes was increased, and a number of disease-promoting genes were shut off.

More recently, another study demonstrated how diets high in omega-6 fats (remember these are found in vegetable oil—particularly corn oil, safflower oil, and sunflower oil) led to unfavorable changes in the genes. These changes were actually passed on to subsequent generations and increased the risk of cancer. This raises the possibility that you could pass on poor genetics to your kids based solely on your actions.

Another recent study looked at people who carry a gene known as FTO, which increases the risk of obesity. People who carry this gene can silence it simply by exercising. Obesity, even for those with an increased genetic risk of obesity, is not a foregone conclusion.

Want more solid proof? Eating fruits and vegetables can dampen the potentially negative effects of a gene associated with heart disease. Even a week of sleep deprivation altered the activity of over seven hundred genes, including those associated with obesity and heart disease, for the worse. (I'll be discussing the crucial importance of adequate sleep for maintaining a healthy weight in Chapter 13.)

All of this strongly suggests that we can exert a great deal more control over our genetics—which genes are turned on or off—and therefore our health outcomes than we had perhaps realized. The undisputed fact is that the basic genetics of the human race have not changed over the last few decades, but the average weight of our population has. Obesity may have a genetic element, but our genes don't change rapidly. Our environment is the problem.

GUT BACTERIA

An immense number of bacteria—about 100 trillion of them—naturally live in your intestinal tract. Most people have over two hundred different bacteria species in their gut. They're supposed to be there because they carry out a number of essential functions for you. Among other things, bacteria in your intestines produce vitamin K (needed for blood clotting) and help break down and digest carbohydrates. The type and quantity of bacteria in the gut work with your body in ways that can prevent or promote weight gain and disease. Recent research suggests that when the gut bacteria population is altered in some way—by taking antibiotics, say—weight gain or weight loss may occur. One bacterium called *Methanobrevibacter smithii*, for example, is found in much higher numbers in overweight people. Because this bacterium helps digest the carbohydrates found in dietary fiber, it's possible that having a lot of it means that you digest dietary fiber more thoroughly. Instead of passing through you, the fiber is digested and releases extra calories that lead to weight gain.

Ordinarily, all of those different bacteria species jostle with each other for space in your gut and keep each other in check. Sometimes, however, the gut bacteria population is altered and gets out of balance. Many factors, ranging from stress to illness to medication to toxins and the type of food we eat, can upset the balance. In the short term, the result of an imbalance could be diarrhea or gas. In the long term, an imbalance can cause weight gain or loss.

Many of the initial studies on gut bacteria were done in animal populations. For instance, mice that were deficient in a particular protein that regulates intestinal bacteria were found to develop low-grade inflammation and insulin resistance. This caused them to eat about 10 percent more food and weigh about 20 percent more than those that didn't have the altered intestinal bacteria. Other studies have found that changes in the natural bacteria can also affect the key hormones from the gut that are necessary for weight control.

Observational studies in humans also show similar relationships to obesity. A recent human study showed that antibiotics, which kill bad bacteria and also the good gut bacteria, changed the levels of the gut hormones that tell us if we're hungry or full. More than 50 years ago, a study of Navy recruits who were given antibiotics showed that they gained twice as much weight as Navy recruits who were given a placebo (sugar pill). They ate more because they didn't feel full. Obese people who lose weight or who have gastric bypass surgery have changes in their gut bacteria population—the balance starts to resemble that of lean people.

The converse is also true. Some studies show that changing the makeup of the gut bacteria by taking prebiotics (nondigestible carbohydrates that stimulate the growth of bacteria) or probiotics (supplements containing good bacteria) may reverse weight gain. Probiotics may also help restore a healthy balance of gut bacteria after taking antibiotics or being sick with an intestinal illness.

Probiotics are naturally found in active culture yogurt and naturally fermented foods such as sauerkraut, sour pickles, and miso. They're also available in pills as supplements.

You can see how important it is to keep a desirable population of bacteria in your gut. To do so, take antibiotics only when necessary. If you must take them, take a course of probiotics after each course of antibiotics. Eat a diet that includes fermented foods and avoids both sugar and an overabundance of saturated fat. Choose low-fat yogurt, for example, instead of sweetened, full-fat versions. If you feel you are not doing as well as you should, take a high-quality probiotic supplement that contains both lactobacillus and bifidobacterium species to help get your gut bacteria back to a healthy balance.

SOCIAL ASPECTS OF WEIGHT LOSS

Another possible contributor to the obesity problem is that there may be a social aspect to gaining weight. A study published in the prestigious *New England Journal of Medicine* suggests that gaining weight is "socially contagious." The study showed that social ties, even outside of family members, played a strong role in weight gain. For instance, a subject's chances of becoming obese increased 57 percent if a friend also gained weight; if a spouse gained weight, the risk of obesity went up 37 percent. These relationships are obviously not genetic, so the social aspect is the culprit. Ordinarily, a normal-weight person has a 2 percent chance of becoming obese in any given year. Based on this study, that number increases by 0.4 percent with each obese contact that person has. On that basis, having just five obese social contacts doubles the baseline risk of being obese yourself. This finding held true even if the friend lived hundreds of miles away, so it's more than just hanging out with people who have similar eating habits.

The researchers in this particular study proposed that the results may simply demonstrate our evolving ideas about what an acceptable weight is. For example, if you go back 25 years or more and look at the "fat" characters in TV shows and movies, in many cases, they wouldn't be considered as heavy by today's standards. Regardless of the research theory, the bottom line is that we tend to spend time with people we like and whom we have the most in common with. We're influenced by and influence those we socialize with. We need to consider whether that modified perception is helping us achieve our health and wellness goals or not.

What if your friends and family aren't supportive of your goals? Janine, one of my patients, was very successful with her weight-loss efforts. On a weekend road trip with her daughter and her daughter's friend, she stuck firmly to her eating plan. Whenever they stopped for gas, the daughter and friend would get candy or some other junk food, but Janine would snack on the fruit she had brought with her. She got a lot of grief for not giving in and eating junk food, but Janine was seeing success with her new lifestyle and was determined not to get sidetracked. During the trip, she realized something that was greatly helpful to her. She told me she realized she was being pressured to make bad choices because her daughter and friend were feeling uncomfortable about their *own* choices compared to hers. This insight gave Janine the self-confidence to take their comments in stride, stick to her own decision, and avoid any ripples in their relationship.

EVERYTHING IN PERSPECTIVE

As a nation, Americans are obsessed with the subject of weight. Yet the results don't match the degree of mental woe that many people experience when they try to address their weight issues. I understand all the reasons for wanting and needing to keep weight under control, but the focus seems to be in the wrong place. Everything seems geared toward managing the weight itself, and not on the bigger picture of achieving a healthy way of life and having the weight fall into place as a result of that. When you focus solely on the scales, your weight becomes a foreboding, negative influence in your life. Small successes or failures are magnified, leading to short-term behaviors that are unsustainable. Eventually, many will feel helpless and give up. Besides, you could be normal weight and be just as unhealthy as those who are carrying too much weight. Focusing solely on a number on the scale is not a good measure for health and well-being.

Scrap the scale. The focus should be on health, not weight. Following the recommendations in this book, the YOU+ app, and the website *will* help you achieve significant weight loss if you need to, but not by dieting or focusing on the scale. Instead, your weight loss will follow on the coattails of knowledge, efficiency, feeling better, and being more energetic. We eat for many more reasons than just our weight. Eating is one of life's simplest pleasures, and yet many of the diet fads people follow ignore this basic reality. They focus instead on weight loss at the cost of eliminating whole categories of food, such as certain fruits, vegetables, grains, adequate fiber, and meat.

At the same time, I believe that many of the official government dietary recommendations, such as those found at Choose-MyPlate.gov, miss the boat. They look at health parameters such as saturated fat or calcium consumption, but they ignore the impact of physical activity on how food is utilized by the body. Doesn't it stand to reason that what you eat could affect you differently, depending on the type and intensity of exercise you do? Or if you don't really exercise at all? A lot of data supports this, but it hasn't yet made it into the mainstream nutritional recommendations. When you pick up a newspaper or magazine and read about one kind of diet being better than another, it probably has been studied in the vacuum of weight loss only, without any regard for differences in, or pairings with, physical activity. In this book, the YOU+ app, and the website, you'll learn how to match your diet to your activity level for maximum insulin efficiency and maximum energy. Weight loss and a more vibrant life will be the side benefits.

CHAPTER 5
THE YOU+ FOOD AND DRINK PLAN

FOR A HEALTHY LIFESTYLE to be sustainable, it's important to keep things simple. People just won't stick to something long-term if it requires them to think too much, spend too much time, or count grams of this or grams of that at every meal. People also won't stick to something that requires them to eat foods that they don't like, or makes them feel hungry all the time, or limits the foods they can choose from to the point where it becomes boring or they feel deprived. The YOU+ approach, already successfully used by many of my patients, incorporates the simple principles that you have just read about. Now that you understand them, you can follow the program without having to think too much about the details and science that sit behind it. The YOU+ method allows you to choose foods you enjoy to fulfill the recommendations for maximum success.

FOOD ON THE YOU+ METHOD

The basic principle of the YOU+ plan, as explained in this book, in the app, and on the website, is to use your eyes. You don't need to obsessively measure out your food or constantly count up the calories or fat grams. All you need to follow the YOU+ plan is a simple system for estimating the proportions of your food with reasonable accuracy. You don't have to even think about the size of your portions—stick to the ratio guidelines I'll describe below, and you can even go back for seconds.

Here's how it works. When you choose your foods at a meal, the size of the protein portion of the meal should be approximately the size of your hand, from your wrist to your fingertips. The size of the total carbohydrate (starch) portion should also be approximately the size of your hand. If you steadily follow this 1:1 ratio of protein to starch, you will naturally take in fewer calories over time without feeling deprived. You'll feel satisfied by each meal, but you won't overeat.

Even though you're taking in somewhat fewer calories, the reason this ratio works well isn't just because you're eating less. It works because it gradually alters your production of gut hormones. You will begin to regulate your appetite naturally as your gut hormones get better at telling your brain you're full.

The YOU+ program isn't a calorie-counting plan. In fact, forget all the calorie-counting books and calculators—forget the angst they cause. The YOU+ method works by using your own body's natural controls and by improving insulin efficiency. Remember, when your leptin is no longer blocked by higher-than-necessary insulin levels, it will reach your brain as it should. The message that you're full will naturally help you to control your appetite, feel more satisfied, and be more active and energetic.

For people who want to lose weight more quickly, or for people who have a hard time losing weight, the ratio of protein to starch needs to be modified to cut back on the starch side. In that case, the protein portion should be the size of your whole hand and the starch portion should be roughly the size of your palm. The ratio becomes 2:1, or roughly twice as much protein as starch.

Although I recommend your hand as a convenient way to judge your portion size, it's the ratio, not the size, that counts. In other words, if your protein portion is smaller than your hand, make sure your starch portion is as well to keep the ratio the same.

If you decide you want a second helping, wait at least twenty minutes from the time you started your meal. You might not feel hungry by that point because your digestive hormones will have kicked in and told your brain you've had enough to eat. The hunger hormone ghrelin, for example, stops being produced once your stomach is full, but it takes about twenty minutes for the change in ghrelin production to happen and be registered by your brain. If you're still hungry after twenty minutes, it's definitely OK to eat some more. Just keep the relative portion sizes the same, even if you choose a smaller amount.

The 1:1 or 2:1 ratio of protein to starch stimulates your natural gut hormones to produce a sense of fullness and satisfaction from less food. Add in the fiber from vegetables and fruits and you'll feel truly sated. You won't be hungry, you'll naturally eat less at each meal, and you'll stay satisfied for longer. The YOU+ method is very helpful for cutting back on between-meal snacking because you just don't feel like eating for longer after a meal.

CHOOSING YOUR FOODS

On the YOU+ plan, fruits and vegetables aren't counted as starches. In fact, although at least one fruit or vegetable needs to be included with every meal, they're not counted at all—eat as much of them as you wish. There's no need to think about ratios or portion sizes. (Juices with sugar added don't count as a fruit or vegetable. Avoid these whenever possible.) The inclusion of a fruit or vegetable with every meal is a vital part of making the YOU+ method work.

WHAT'S IN YOUR FOOD?

For our purposes, I define starches as carbohydrate foods that break down into glucose when they're digested. So, starchy foods include bread of all kinds, pasta, rice, and other foods made from grains, such as couscous and tortillas. Potatoes are also starchy foods. On the YOU+ plan, corn kernels are a veggie. Even though they're technically a starchy grain, corn kernels are also high in fiber and full of vitamins and other nutrients—they act much more like vegetables than starches on your blood sugar.

Sugary foods also count on the starch side of the ratio, but they should be limited in your eating plan. Added sugars are detrimental to your health because they break down differently in the body when they're digested (check back to Chapter 3). The sugar is much more likely to end up as fat in your liver and on your waistline. Food with added sugars—cookies, for example—are also likely to be high in carbohydrates that aren't balanced by protein.

When calculating your starch intake in relation to your protein intake, remember to consider *all* the starch eaten during your meal. For example, if you eat a roll with dinner, then you must balance that with less starch elsewhere in your meal. You might choose a smaller portion of mashed potatoes, for example. Or, if you know your favorite mashed potatoes are on the menu, you could skip the dinner roll and eat more of the potatoes.

Whenever possible, choose a whole grain or whole food for your starch—that way you get all of the natural nutrients in the food, including the hunger-killing fiber, and avoid the added sugars that are found in some 80 percent of processed foods. Opt for brown rice instead of white rice, a baked potato instead of french fries, whole wheat pasta instead of semolina pasta, and so on. Expand your horizons a bit with alternatives to wheat-based foods—look into other grains, such as quinoa and amaranth. Beans or sweet potatoes make a good alternative to white potatoes (more about beans later on in this chapter).

Whenever possible, your protein choice should be fish or skinless poultry. Try to limit lean pork and beef to about one-third or less of your protein intake across a week. Look for cuts labeled round or loin; for hamburger meat, select 90 to 95 percent lean.

If you eat red meat for more than about a third of your protein intake over a week, you could end up getting too much iron from your food. You could also end up making your gut bacteria produce too much of an artery-clogging compound called TMAO as they digest the amino acid carnitine found in red meat.

Also try to limit processed meats such as bacon and hot dogs—these foods contain large amounts of artificial flavorings and other chemical additives that are best avoided. Remember, just one daily portion of processed meat is enough to raise your risk of deadly disease by 42 percent.

Choose lean proteins that are baked, sautéed, broiled, steamed, or grilled. Avoid breaded or battered proteins (bread crumbs for crunchiness are fine). Also avoid deep-fried proteins (which are often breaded or battered).

Milk, cheese, and dairy products count as protein choices. A milk or yogurt serving is 8 ounces (1 cup)—consider that amount as equivalent to the size of your hand. I suggest aiming for two to three servings of dairy foods each day as part of your protein/starch ratio. Avoid dairy foods with added sugar, such as chocolate milk and yogurt with sweetened fruit.

Eggs also count as lean protein. Contrary to popular belief, eggs do not raise your cholesterol. This has been validated by dozens of studies, all of which found that daily consumption of one or more eggs did not increase the risk of heart disease or stroke among healthy people. Eggs are inexpensive, easy to prepare, and a near-perfect protein source. They're also a great source of many vitamins, minerals, and antioxidants. There's no reason to avoid them. Consider two eggs, however they're prepared, as being the size of your hand.

What about foods such as beans and nuts, which are good mix of protein and carbohydrates? If you eat beans along with a protein source—baked beans with your grilled steak, for instance—think of the beans as a vegetable. Their carbohydrate content is counterbalanced by their high fiber content, just as with corn. But beans are also an excellent source of protein by themselves. If you're eating them as the main part of your meal, think of them as your protein portion. In that case, ignore their carbohydrates and adjust your intake of other carbohydrates to keep your ratio in balance.

Although nuts contain some carbohydrates, they're also high in protein. When it comes to your protein-carbohydrate ratio at a meal, think of nuts as a protein with a nice fiber bonus, no matter what else you're eating. Ignore their carbohydrates and adjust the carbohydrates in your meal to keep your ratio in balance.

If you don't eat meat or animal foods, beans and nuts are important to you on the YOU+ plan because they become an important source of protein in your diet. If that's the case for you, you can largely ignore the carbohydrates in these foods and focus on the protein. To stick with a good ratio for beans and nuts, imagine your fist as your portion size—this works out to about 1 cup in volume. If the beans or nuts are your main protein at that meal, you will probably want to have one to two "fists" as your portion. (The YOU+ app and website have more information on good protein sources for people who don't eat much or any meat and other animal products.)

Nuts are an excellent source of protein—and they also contain healthy omega-3 and omega-9 fatty acids. Nuts are also an excellent source of vitamins (especially folate and vitamin E), minerals (especially magnesium), and fiber. A number of studies have shown that people who eat a lot of nuts have a lower risk of heart disease. For a snack, a protein portion of nuts is the amount in a large handful, or about two tablespoons of a nut butter.

PACKAGED AND RESTAURANT FOODS

Many packaged and restaurant foods are prepared in combination, so you need to look carefully to determine the protein/ starch ratio. Most food packages have a picture of the food on them, so you can easily take a look and estimate the ratio. What if you're in a restaurant? You can't always estimate a ratio by looking at your entree. You'll just have to aim for a reasonable estimate. Start by deciding if the food is predominantly protein or carbohydrate, and use whichever you choose as the basis for your ratio. Lasagna, for instance, contains meat and cheese, which are proteins, but it's mostly pasta, which is a starch. Your portion of lasagna would therefore count as more starch than protein in the calculation of your ratio. Most pasta dishes, and a lot of pizzas, count as carbohydrate. On the other hand, protein is the main feature of tuna salad, and therefore would count as a protein in the calculation of the ratio.

If the food is in a package—a prepared frozen meal, for instance—look carefully at it to visualize the protein-carbohydrate ratio. You can check how accurate your estimate is by looking at the nutrition facts label to see how the protein and starch stack up in grams. Reading food labels is a useful skill for making good choices. If you look at the labels on your favorite foods, you'll quickly get a good sense of the protein-carbohydrates ratio.

Most people don't read past the fat content on a label. Because you're now reading the label more carefully, you're getting much more information than the average person. You'll see, for instance, that a surprising number of packaged meals have added sugar.

What if the meal you're served has only one predominant feature and it's in the form of carbohydrate? Let's go back to that lasagna, which is more starch than protein and sends the ratio in the wrong direction. If there are no other choices at the meal to fill out the opposite side of the ratio, it's still OK to eat the lasagna. Just make up for it by the end of the day or the start of the next. That should quickly get you back to approximating the desired 1:1 or 2:1 ratio. You could just eliminate starch at the next meal, for example. That's not really hard to do. You could have lasagna for lunch and make up for it at dinner by skipping the starch and sticking to grilled protein of some kind, vegetables, and salad.

THE BIGGER PICTURE

The ratio at any one meal is less important than achieving the overall protein-starch ratio across the day or even across a few days. When you can't get a good protein-starch balance at a single meal, you can almost always manage the other part of the equation, which is to have a vegetable or fruit with every meal. You could easily order a green salad along with the lasagna, for example.

A meal plan needs to be practical and doable—and it needs to acknowledge that you're not always perfect. A meal plan without dessert isn't any fun, which means it isn't doable. I encourage you to eat dessert in the form of fresh fruit. But to make the plan truly doable, I also encourage you to eat an appropriately sized dessert (such as a scoop of ice cream or medium-sized piece of cake) once a week in addition to your cheat day if you choose (I'll explain about cheat days later in this chapter). Having a sweet dessert more often than once or twice a week can kick-start sugar cravings, which are very hard to resist. The rest of the week, choose fresh fruit as your dessert. Count a sweet dessert as a starch in your overall meal ratio. So, if you want to have a brownie for dessert, skip the rice pilaf with your main course.

For those times when you simply must have something sweet, try a few squares of high-quality dark chocolate, or something equally small and delicious. You'll quench the desire without affecting your ratio much.

BEVERAGES ON THE YOU+ METHOD

The best choices of beverages on the YOU+ method are any kind of tea (iced or hot), water, milk, and coffee. Sugared drinks— soda, sweetened fruit drinks, sports drinks—create additional health problems beyond their empty calories, and should be avoided as much as possible. Sugar-free drinks have their own issues as well. (Check back to Chapter 3 for more on this.) If, despite all their drawbacks, you can't get yourself to give up diet drinks, then at least try to limit them as much as you can.

Alcohol can throw even the best-laid health plan into disarray. Let me be clear—I am not a teetotaler. I enjoy a good glass of wine with dinner, and I wouldn't begrudge you something similar. I'm not suggesting you give up alcohol altogether. Based on my experience with many patients over the years, however, there is little doubt that excessive alcohol makes it difficult for people to meet their fitness goals. The problem with alcohol is that because it is metabolized in the liver in much the same way as fructose, it is destined to be stored as fat.

Once you realize the impact of too much alcohol, often everything else will fall into place. Certainly many of my patients have experienced this.

Too much alcohol can mean different things to different people. One example is Susan, a 70-year-old patient who was seemingly doing everything right. She went to the gym a few times a week, ate pretty much the right foods, and slept well. She was frustrated that she couldn't reach her weight goal. We decided that she should stop the one glass of wine she had every night. We talked about how alcohol is metabolized in the liver and turned into fat. I used the analogy of a sculptor adding to a statue—but instead of clay, it was alcohol adding fat to her body. By eliminating the daily intake of sugar and alcohol that were in the wine, Susan began to lose a couple of extra pounds every month. She reached her goal weight sooner than we had hoped.

Evaluate yourself honestly to see if this is an area holding you back. Some studies suggest a daily drink might help prevent heart disease. This may be true, but I believe it needs to be looked at in the context of the overall health and diet picture. If you are carrying more weight than you should, eliminating or significantly reducing your intake of alcohol could yield considerable benefits on your health and fitness.

CHEAT DAY

I'm not perfect (as evidenced by my doughnut episode), and I certainly don't expect you to be either! On the YOU+ method, you get to indulge yourself with a "cheat day" one half-day each week. On that day, you can splurge and have things that you wouldn't regularly have during the rest of the week. Maybe it's ice cream, maybe it's pancakes, pie, pizza, ribs, or a plate of spaghetti. Whatever it is, by splurging just this one half-day a week, you give yourself permission to enjoy favorite foods that you've largely avoided the rest of the week. Half a day of indulgence is enjoyable, yet it's not long enough to undo all the good you've done for yourself by following the YOU+ plan the rest of the week.

A cheat day also does something else that's extremely important. It helps you manage temptation. I don't want you to think you can never again have something you really like—that's too difficult for anyone over the long term. When faced with a tempting food, it's much easier to say "I'll wait until Saturday" (or whatever day you pick).

Cheat days are flexible. They don't have to be the same day every week, but they must be *only* once a week—otherwise, you defeat the purpose. Many of my patients time their cheat days for regular events, such as the weekly staff dinner, poker night, or Sunday dinner with the family. If you know a big celebration or holiday is coming up, try to have it coincide with your cheat day.

HOW OFTEN SHOULD YOU EAT?

The standard recommendation nutritionists give for increasing your metabolism is eating smaller, more frequent meals. This is supposed to keep you from feeling hungry, even as it speeds up your weight loss. As it turns out, this is another diet myth that simply isn't true.

In fact, most people who eat six small meals a day end up taking in more calories than those who eat three larger meals. Lots of studies show this. One compared people who took in the same number of calories, either from two large meals a day or six smaller meals. Even though their caloric intake was the same, the people who ate only twice a day had more weight loss. A study in the *British Journal of Nutrition* echoes other studies in showing that eating more frequent meals does *not* cause a significant increase metabolism to counter the increased intake of food. Other investigators have shown that although eating fewer than three meals a day can make us feel less satiated, eating more than three meals a day doesn't make us feel more satiated.

Looking at the data, it would seem that eating three meals daily does the most to satisfy your hunger throughout the day— probably because of the effects of the gut hormones you are now familiar with—while promoting greater weight loss. If you follow the YOU+ eating plan, your daily three meals can be as large as you want, so long as you stick to the carbohydrate-protein ratio. Three meals a day with the right ratio does a lot to reduce between-meal hunger and the urge to snack.

If you do get hungry between meals, try to stick to snacks that are either protein sources or fruits and vegetables. In fact, you can eat as many fruits and vegetables as you want, whenever you want them. For your protein snacks, aim for cheese, yogurt (without loads of sugar), nuts, baked chicken legs, soft- or hard-boiled eggs (I soft boil some ahead so they are always available in the refrigerator), and the like. If you want something starchy, popcorn is a good choice.

One of your three daily meals must be breakfast. People who skip breakfast have been shown to have more weight gain and also worse health—they're more likely to have heart disease, for instance. This may be because skipping breakfast leads to higher insulin levels later in the day. Those higher insulin levels have all the bad effects we've discussed, including blocking the effect of leptin, which makes you feel more hungry and be less active.

A PRACTICAL EXAMPLE

So what will the YOU+ plan look like for you on a typical day? Let's look at what you'd choose to eat while getting together with friends at a summer cookout.

Your meat choices at the cookout are likely to be something like burgers, barbequed chicken, and hot dogs. Skip the hot dogs—processed meats just aren't good for you. There's a huge nutritional difference between the effects of unprocessed meats and processed meats. Let's say you choose to have a hamburger. The bun is a starch, and it's probably at least as big as the burger (protein), so you're pretty close to the 1:1 ratio. If you're aiming more for a 2:1 ratio, you're still close—you can easily accommodate the mismatch elsewhere in the meal.

For a side dish, your choices might be grilled corn on the cob, baked beans, potato salad, and green salad. What should you go for? The baked beans are a good option. The potato salad is a starch, but if you've already met your ratio of starch to protein with that hamburger bun, you should definitely skip this. If you really love potato salad, though, you could skip the bun on your burger, or go with the chicken, and still be at your proper protein-starch ratio. The grilled corn on the cob should be seen as just another vegetable, so it's fine to have it—or even more than one serving of it. You can also have as much of the green salad (and the sliced tomatoes, coleslaw, three-bean salad, and other vegetables) as you want.

What about that peach cobbler that looks so good? If this is your cheat day or the one other day a week you have dessert, enjoy it while still staying on the plan. Forgo the other starch options of the bun and potato salad and have a piece of the cobbler relative to the size of the burger or chicken you choose. Because fruits and vegetables are always free in the ratio, you can also have as much watermelon and other fruit as you can eat for dessert.

This way of choosing foods keeps you in control and allows you to make choices between foods that you like in order to fulfill the ratio of protein to starch. It also gives you a high degree of freedom so you won't feel restricted. If you can make it comfortably through a simple backyard barbeque, you'll have the confidence to go into almost any situation and make choices that are best suited to your goals. Clearly, the choices you're provided with aren't always going to be ideal, but you can make the most of whatever situation you're in. No one will ever need to know you're even following a plan.

EATING OUT

My patients sometimes worry about following a healthy eating plan when they're in a social setting or eating out. Often we don't want to draw attention to our dietary changes and as a result can easily decide to go off the plan to avoid embarrassment. This is especially true when eating out—and nearly one in four meals eaten in the United States comes from a restaurant. Eating out a lot can make it very difficult to control your weight. In addition, you have no way of knowing the calorie content of many restaurant meals. If you did, it would shock you—they're often much higher than you would expect based on what you cook for yourself at home. Take Applebee's, for example. The food tastes great, but it can blow your eating plan right out of the water. The fish and chips dish at Applebee's is 1,700 calories; the spinach and artichoke dip appetizer is 1,320 calories. Think a salad is a safer bet? Not necessarily. The full-size Moroccan chicken salad at California Pizza Kitchen is 1,500 calories. When the calorie counts are that high—almost a full day's worth in just one dish—trying to figure out the carbohydrate-protein ratio won't help you as much. You just have to make the best choices under the circumstances. Here's where the YOU+ app is extremely valuable. Use it to find the best choices, based on the overall nutritional picture of a dish, not just the calories. The app lists the dishes at popular restaurants across five hundred thousand locations nationally. Tell the app what restaurant you're at and the best menu choices, based on the carb-protein ratio and other nutritional considerations, pop up.

Making an effort to eat more meals at home (or taking your meals with you) is an important part of achieving your health and fitness goals. When you prepare your own food, you can control what you eat. The reality, though, is that in our busy society, we will still eat a lot of meals away from home despite our best efforts.

In addition to striving for a good protein-starch ratio, many other good strategies for eating out can help you keep your goals from being derailed. Try them.

- Don't be afraid to make special requests. The restaurant wants you back as a customer and will make an effort to satisfy almost any reasonable request. Today, asking for extra vegetables or a salad instead of fries isn't even really a special request. Ditto for asking for a bunless burger.

- When you first sit down, and are most hungry and tempted, the waiter will ask you if you want an appetizer. That increases the restaurant's sales, but it also increases your waistline. A lot of restaurant appetizers, like deep-fried onions or artichoke and spinach dip, are health-busters. If those are the only choices, just say no. But if you're really hungry, or if everyone else is ordering an appetizer and you don't want to stand out, look for healthy choices, such as grilled shrimp. You can always ask for a salad even if it's not on the appetizer menu.

- If you choose to have a hamburger on a bun, you have achieved your ratio, which means the fries will upset the balance. Substitute a side salad, vegetable, or fruit for the french fries. You already know this, but sometimes you actually need to do it.

- Avoid foods described as crispy, breaded, fried, au gratin, or stuffed. Go for the ones that are baked, broiled, sautéed, steamed, roasted, or grilled.

- Remember that the bread or chips in the basket count toward the carbohydrate side of the ratio, so go easy on them.

- Ask for sauces, gravies, and dressings on the side. Use them sparingly—in restaurants, these often have added sugar. If a dish is prepared in a broth or reduction, you don't need to have it on the side.

- Take it easy with the cheese. Even though dairy foods have an important part to play in the YOU+ method, the calories at a restaurant can be astronomical. Skipping the cheese is a good way to reduce the excessive calorie counts in restaurant dishes.

- In restaurants, beware of pasta dishes, casseroles, and the like. Again, the calorie counts can be surprisingly high. You can use visual methods to get a good idea of the protein-starch ratio in pasta dishes, but casseroles are much harder to estimate.

AT HOME

It's much easier to make healthy choices at home, even when you're busy and even when you're not much of a cook. Try starting out with just one extra meal at home a week for a few weeks. Once you get the idea, it's easier to then add an additional meal at home the following week, and build up to as many meals at home as are practical for you. Even these small changes will be helpful. You'll feel good about yourself, and you might even learn to cook better and enjoy it more. Eating more meals at home is easier if you keep things simple:

- Plan what to have for the meals at home a week ahead. That way you can get everything you need in just one trip to the grocery store and have it at home. This forward planning will reduce the number of poor choices you make because you don't have healthier ingredients at hand. Good intentions are one thing, but good planning will lead to success. The YOU+ app and website will give you hundreds of delicious ideas that will fit the protein-starch ratio. The app will even help you create shopping lists to take with you to the store.

- Grocery stores now have plenty of healthy prepared items that make meals at home much simpler. Rotisserie chickens, salad bags, prewashed and cut fruits and vegetables, and even prepared vegetable dishes make it very easy to put together a healthy meal with minimal cooking. If even that's too much, look for smart frozen entrees.

- Prepare a large batch of food on the weekend or on your days off work. Eat some that day, save some for later in the week, and freeze some for quick meals in the future.

- Keep fruits, nuts, and other healthy snacks in view. You're much more likely to eat an apple if it's in front of you on the counter than if you have to dig for it in the refrigerator.

- You have to like what you're eating. Don't buy something just because it's "healthy" and then have it sit there and eventually get thrown out because you don't like it. Before you buy it, make sure it really is healthy—junk food made with organic ingredients is still junk food. But do try new things. You may come across new foods you like and that fit well with the YOU+ plan—pumpkin seeds as a snack, for instance.

With all of this in mind, let's take a look at some options for a typical day that will allow you to stick with the YOU+ plan and gain its optimal fitness and health benefits. These are just ideas; you'll find many more on the YOU+ app and website. Mix and match these and other items to meet the guidelines. You can create countless menus that keep the YOU+ principles in mind and are made with the foods you enjoy.

BREAKFAST SUGGESTIONS

- Two eggs, 1 slice whole grain toast, melon or other fruit.

- Oatmeal made with milk instead of water (to increase protein and achieve the 1:1 ratio) and topped with a banana, strawberries, and/or blueberries. If you made the oatmeal with water, you could add a side dish of turkey bacon or sausage or a glass of milk.

- A protein shake made with milk, cocoa powder, banana, a little peanut butter, and a scoop of whey protein powder.

- Two scrambled eggs made with fresh vegetables, such as green peppers, spinach, mushrooms, tomatoes, onions, zucchini, broccoli, or even artichokes. Whole grain English muffin.

- Soft- or hard-boiled egg, whole grain cereal with fruit on top. Add 1 cup of milk to the cereal to get the right protein-starch ratio. For any breakfast that has a lot of starch (cereal, toast, muffin), a glass of milk is an easy way to even out the ratio.

- A European-style breakfast of bread or croissant, with a variety of cheeses and fruit such as grapes or melon. My mother-in-law prepared this on a family trip, and it has really made for a great addition to our breakfast repertoire ever since.

LUNCH SUGGESTIONS

- Chicken or lean beef burrito with salsa and avocado.

- Tuna salad (try it made with a little olive oil and balsamic vinegar instead of mayonnaise) on whole grain crackers with an apple, pear, or grapes.

- Leftovers from the night before or lower-carb frozen entrée.

- Turkey or roast beef sandwich on whole grain bread, along with precut and washed vegetables with hummus dip. Consider having the sandwich on just one slice of bread and adding some whole grain pretzels as a substitute for the bread.

- Salad with grilled chicken or roast beef, tomatoes, green, yellow and red peppers, avocado, a little cheese, and olive oil or canola dressing. Add some yogurt or cottage cheese if no protein is on the salad. For your salad, go beyond iceberg lettuce and try other types of greens, such as arugula, romaine, or red leaf lettuce.

- Hard-boiled egg and a whole-grain pita filled with vegetables and cheddar cheese.

- A cup of lean-meat chili made with beans and a small side salad with olive oil or canola dressing; have a piece of fruit if no salad is available.

- Everyone going out for lunch? Check the menu and make a tasty choice that keeps the YOU+ principles in mind. Even fast-food restaurants have some choices that will leave you feeling good about yourself.

- At lunch, choose milk for your beverage if you need to add protein.

DINNER SUGGESTIONS

- Grilled flank steak marinated in olive oil, chopped garlic, and chipotle peppers; served with baked potato and broccoli.

- Boneless pork chop, brown rice or quinoa, corn, or natural applesauce.

- Sirloin steak, baked sweet potato, green beans, small salad.

- Chicken Marsala with greens sautéed in olive oil or baked squash.

- Salmon grilled on tinfoil with chopped green onions, seasoned salt, and olive oil; baked potato wedges and asparagus.

- Sloppy Joe filling (no bun, eat with a fork), baked beans, and a piece of fruit or a vegetable.

- Tilapia filet with boiled new potatoes and Brussels sprouts oven-roasted with olive oil and balsamic vinegar.

- Grilled chicken breast with a slice of mozzarella cheese melted over it and covered with marinara sauce, bread to be dipped in olive oil with a little Parmesan cheese, spinach salad, grapes.

- Burrito made with lean ground beef, refried beans, onions, taco sauce, and cheese; tortilla chips with guacamole.

- Rotisserie chicken, mashed potatoes, and peas. If you also picked up an angel food cake at the grocery store, have a piece of that with strawberries instead of the potatoes to keep your proper ratio.

These ideas are just a tiny sample of the food choice options available to you through the YOU+ app and website. By following the YOU+ plan, you will naturally reduce your caloric intake without counting them or even really paying any attention to them. At the same time, you'll enjoy your food and won't feel as if you're depriving yourself. You have science on your side; you just need to choose the foods you enjoy to get the job done. When you do, it will be easy for you to make the long-term dietary changes that will help you meet your goals.

CHAPTER 6
VITAL NUTRIENTS

W HEN YOU FIRST HEAR the term "vital nutrients," you might assume that this is a chapter about the food and drink you should consume to get the basic nutrition you need to stay alive: protein, carbohydrates, fats, water, and vitamins and minerals.

Vital nutrients, however, also includes dietary supplements that the body may require for optimal performance. But before we go any further, I want to emphasize that a supplement is only that. It's something to supplement your diet if there is an existing shortfall. Not too many of us in today's world manage to eat the perfect balance of vital nutrients, and, as a result, many of us are a bit low on some important nutrients. Supplements can help make up the difference in the right circumstances.

What supplements are not, however, is a way to get those vital nutrients without eating the right foods. Again, supplements are just that—supplemental—and are never a replacement for trying to eat the right foods. They should be used only as a fallback position to fill any shortfalls or occasional gaps.

We seem to have lost track of that, and I can understand why. This trend began more than a century ago, when medical science first began to isolate active substances in foods, although at first, they weren't really sure what they had found. It wasn't until the 1930s that vitamins—organic substances that are necessary for life and must be obtained from the diet—began to be isolated. Vitamin C, for instance, was discovered in 1931 by Albert Szent-Györgyi; he received the Nobel Prize for his work in 1937. Citrus fruits and many other fruits and vegetables contain vitamin C in abundance. Scurvy, the deficiency disease caused by lack of vitamin C, is easily cured simply by eating foods high in vitamin C. Even so, the natural extension of the discovery of vitamin C was to make it into a supplement. The same approach applied to all the later vitamin and mineral discoveries, to say nothing of all the other substances, such as antioxidants, that play a role in human health.

There was a downside to all the nutritional discoveries. Americans are notoriously busy, rushing from one commitment to the next, and, consequently, an unhealthy assumption developed: "Forget the food. Just take a pill and get what you need (or be 'cured' of some health problem) without the hassle." This message has been repeated by clever marketers for countless substances. And we've bought it hook, line, and sinker, to the point where taking supplements, many of them of dubious value, has become part of our culture.

Do you remember the TV cartoon "The Jetsons"? It was a cartoon about a futuristic twenty-first century family. As well as getting around in flying cars, whole meals were taken in pill form. Thankfully, we haven't reached that vision (yet), but the notions about the value of isolated elements in food abound. Sadly, you can now buy "healthy" soda and "healthy, flavored" water that have been fortified with vitamins. We have really lost sight of some basic truths about our food.

The first basic truth is that systems, both in nature and in our bodies, are far more complex than this simplistic approach to nutrition. In nature, crucial substances such as vitamin C don't occur in isolation. In their natural form, they're combined with many other substances. An orange, for instance, has about 70 milligrams of vitamin C, but it also has large amounts of flavonoids, compounds found in fruits and vegetables that have a wide range of beneficial effects. In fact, an orange has far more flavonoids in it than vitamin C. When you eat an orange, you get the benefits of everything it contains. In spite of modern nutritional science, we don't even know yet what many of those flavonoids do. But doesn't it stand to reason that they have a purpose? That if we take one part out and isolate it, it won't be the same as the original whole?

An interesting study compared a group of people who drank orange juice to those who drank vitamin C-fortified water. Vitamin C levels in both groups increased in measured blood samples, so we know that both groups were absorbing their drink equally. The samples were then exposed to hydrogen peroxide, which is known to cause damage to your cells. The results were significant. Those who drank the juice had a lesser degree of damage than those who drank the fortified water. The implication here is that there are more things involved with the nutrients in our food than just the vitamin C, and that the combination of substances nature provides is always superior.

A recent study compared bone density in women who got most of their calcium from dietary sources to those who got most of it from supplements. Those who got most of their calcium from dietary sources had higher bone densities than the supplement group, even though their total calcium intake from the dietary sources was lower overall. Nature's design wins again.

The simple fact of the matter is that we are probably never going to do it any better than nature does. Our bodies have developed over time to live on what the planet provides *and* in the proportion nature provides it to us. Our bodies recognize all the one-part-per-million sorts of things that science hasn't even discovered yet but are in the foods we eat. The body recognizes just the right mix, in just the right matrix, absorbed in just the right way. There's no way to replicate that to perfection with supplements; no pill can give us the nutrition that's found naturally in our food. It's kind of like having a favorite dish, and then someone gives you a recipe for it. When you make it at home, it's great, but not quite the same. Maybe something wasn't quite right because someone wanted to keep a secret; maybe your oven doesn't heat up in quite the same way, but in any event, you just can't get it exactly right. When it comes to your health, you can't beat Mother Nature.

Because nature doesn't provide us food components in isolation, it's hard to evaluate studies that look only at one particular food component. All too often, studies of nutrients and food yield conflicting results. Garlic is a popular supplement, for example. Taking garlic supplements is said by some to help prevent heart disease and colorectal cancer and to boost the immune system, among other claims. Do the many studies support these claims? Some do, some don't. What many of these studies don't consider is the possibility that things change when they are processed or put into pill form. For example, the amount of allicin (the purported active ingredient in garlic) in a garlic clove diminishes sharply an hour after the clove has been cut and exposed to the air. If the active ingredient diminishes after an hour, won't even less be left after a garlic clove is processed into pill form? All a study can tell you is if the processed product has any benefit—not if fresh garlic, which contains much more than just allicin, has the same benefit or is even better.

This paradox is true for many other food components isolated into supplements. Manufacturers say that studies support their claims, but remember that you just can't beat getting something in its real, fresh form. While you might hear conflicting things about the benefits of the anthocyanins in blueberries, have you ever read that a blueberry isn't good for you?

The best way to make sure you are getting the full nutritional value of what you eat is to get the food in its whole form. I don't mean buying it at the grocery chain of the same name. I mean eating a food in its intact natural state, before nutrients are stripped away or altered by additives and processing. The term "whole" generally applies to fruits, vegetables, and whole grains, but I extend that meaning to include meats, eggs, fish, and poultry in their natural form as well. By this, as an example, I mean eating boneless skinless chicken breasts, not processed chicken nuggets.

WATER

One nutrient is the most important of all, although it's not commonly thought of as a nutrient at all. It's water. Every function of every system in your body depends on water—in fact, water is the body's main ingredient, making up around 60 percent of our weight. Water is involved in processes from moistening the eyes to preventing constipation to carrying nutrients to expelling toxins. We can survive weeks to months without food, but only days without water.

How much water do we need to drink every day to be healthy? You probably think it's eight 8-ounce glasses, or about two quarts. That's the rule of thumb that's repeated everywhere, even though there's not very much evidence to support it. The 8 x 8 rule, for instance, doesn't take into account the water you get from foods such as fruits and vegetables, which are mostly water, and from other foods such as soup, and beverages such as coffee. It also doesn't take into account your activity level, environment, or body size.

Because even mild dehydration (just 1 percent) can be harmful, the answers to these questions are important. Two of the most common complaints I hear in my medical practice are lack of energy and overactive appetite. Surprisingly, lack of adequate water intake is often a contributing cause. Dehydration make you feel tired, sleepy, and lacking in energy. The brain can perceive thirst as hunger—so instead of drinking something, you eat something, which can lead to taking in a lot of excess calories.

So, let's draw a distinction between the amount of fluid required for minimum health and the amount for optimal health.

The eight glasses a day advice isn't really based on current science. This amount was derived from an idea in 1945 that we should drink 1 milliliter of water for every calorie consumed. If this was accurate, our water requirements today would be significantly more than they were back then. Our average daily calorie intake is now well above the approximately 1900 calories per day it was in 1945. This hypothesis also doesn't factor in the water contained in the foods we eat. For many folks, this accounts for about 20 percent of their average daily fluid intake. Although the 8 x 8 view has been scientifically abandoned, it's still cited as the gold standard.

The reality is that most people get at least the minimum amount of water they need because our thirst mechanism is very finely honed. In other words, we drink when we're thirsty, and that's usually enough to maintain things at an acceptable level, at least from a minimum standard viewpoint. For optimal health, however, we need to look at other variables and be more aware of our need for water to achieve a better level of fitness.

For a start, as we get older, that finely tuned thirst mechanism may not be as finely tuned as it once was. Older people often don't feel as thirsty and don't drink enough. They can get dehydrated more easily, especially in hot weather. At any age, when you exercise at the level needed to optimize your health, your hydration needs also increase.

According to the Institute of Medicine (the folks who set recommended daily allowances), outside of the water in the foods we eat, men should consume about 100 ounces of fluid each day and women about 72 ounces each day to be certain to meet their hydration needs. It has been my experience that people who meet these hydration levels just seem to do better in meeting their fitness and health goals.

Sarah, one my patients, was doing a pretty good job of following the YOU+ nutritional and exercise guidelines I gave her. She was feeling happy about wearing smaller-sized clothes, but her energy levels was still low in spite of adequate rest and her improved fitness level. Low energy was prompting her to eat sugary foods for their quick rush, but sugary foods, in turn, were causing her to lose some of the progress she had made. In the end, the extra sugar wasn't making her feel more energetic, either. We went through her daily routine, looking for what might be sapping Sarah's energy. We quickly realized that her fluid intake was suboptimal. She just wasn't drinking enough, to the point where she was mildly dehydrated all the time. Sarah had a busy schedule and often just didn't have the time or awareness to make sure she drank enough over the course of the day. When she made getting enough to drink a priority, she quickly noticed that her energy was better. To help remind her to drink, Sarah bought a colorful reusable water bottle and kept it on her desk so she would be constantly reminded to drink from it.

The science is still murky regarding water intake as a way to help with weight control. Some studies have shown that drinking a couple of cups of water before eating a meal cuts down on appetite and leads to more weight loss, but others haven't shown much effect. I've found with my patients that drinking water before a meal does help with weight loss, so I recommend it, particularly to those who need an energy boost or have hit a plateau in their weight loss. Of course, on hot days or in very dry weather, aim to drink more than usual.

WHAT SHOULD WE DRINK?

Earlier, I explained about the dangers of the sugar in soda, sports drinks, energy drinks, and sweetened fruit juices and other beverages. I also explained how artificial sweeteners in diet drinks have their own drawbacks, including weight gain. I'm not going to say that I never have a diet soda because I do, so I don't expect you to abstain forever, either. But diet drinks really need to be the smallest possible percentage of what you drink. What does that leave as our choices for getting enough fluid? The answer to that can be gleaned from Grand Island, Nebraska.

Grand Island is a wonderful American small town, and not just because my wife grew up there. Despite its diminutive size, Grand Island's labor market has led to significant diversity, which is reflected in its restaurants. From Sudanese to Salvadoran, the range would rival any block in New York City. However, it is at one of its oldest, distinctly American venues that the answer can be found—the Coney Island lunchroom. Walking into Coney Island is like having a flashback in time. Menu boards from the 1930s are still on the walls, and Gus, the proprietor, can sometimes still be seen working behind the counter. Reminiscent of a time before soda, added sugars, and diet drinks were king, the old-style menu board offers coffee, tea, iced tea, and milk. Although considered by many as relics from a bygone era, these options also represent the modern answer for what to drink. The lion's share of your fluid intake should be plain water, but just drinking water can be a little dull, and it's unrealistic to think that's all you'll ever drink. Coffee, tea, iced tea, and milk therefore provide a welcome addition to the YOU+ plan.

Often, people are surprised by these recommendations because of the caffeine in tea and coffee. While it's true that caffeine has a mild diuretic effect, depleting fluid from your body by making you urinate more, you have to drink a lot of it to notice. It takes four average cups of coffee or ten average cups of tea to get enough caffeine to counteract the benefits of the fluid intake. To help you meet your daily hydration needs while still enjoying caffeinated beverages, drink up to three 8-ounce cups of coffee or six 12-ounce servings of unsweetened iced tea every day. If you do want to limit caffeine, opt for decaffeinated coffee or tea or choose herbal tea instead.

FLUID AND EXERCISE

Exercise increases fluid loss through sweating and faster breathing, so it's important to compensate for the loss effectively. That basically means drinking more plain water. If you follow the exercise recommendations in this book and the YOU+ app and website, you won't need any fluid replacement from sports drinks. The extra ingredients in a sports drink—mostly salt, sugar, and potassium—are only needed if you engage in bouts of high-intensity exercise lasting more than an hour. There are exceptions, such as exercising in hot or humid weather, where you sweat a lot more than usual. Most of the time, however, if you have a sports drinks after moderate-intensity exercise of less than an hour, you will simply be replacing the calories you just burned during your workout! A 32-ounce sports drink contains about 200 calories from sugar. Sometimes carbohydrates are beneficial in exercise training (I'll discuss this further in Chapter 12), but for optimal health—not elite-level sports performance—sports drinks aren't necessary. Advertisers are very good at convincing us otherwise, but science doesn't support the claims. If you start your workout normally hydrated, all you need to do is replace the fluid you lose when exercising. That fluid doesn't need to contain extra calories or anything else— stick to plain water.

The replacement amount will vary based on how much you sweat and how hot it is when you exercise. For most people, 8 to 24 ounces (one to three cups) of water per hour will take care of the replacement need. Shorter exercise sessions generally require proportionately less fluid intake; if you exercise for half an hour, you would probably require half as much water.

Just as with total daily intake, women generally require less fluid replacement than men following exercise. In the end, male or female, if you drink at least 16 ounces of water within a short time of completing an hour-long workout, you've probably done enough to rehydrate. Because hydration is so important, however, try to drink during your workout instead of waiting until you're done. Aim for 8 to 16 ounces during a half-hour exercise session and count it toward your replacement needs. The more you drink during your workout, the less you need to drink later.

If you're an unusually heavy sweater, you may require more water, perhaps up to a fourth cup or a total of 32 ounces per hour for replacement. If you want to be more precise, a quick way to check is to weigh yourself before and after an exercise session to see how much weight you really lose from sweating. Every pound you lose should be replaced by 16 ounces of water, whether you're male or female. After you've measured yourself a few times, the results can serve as your guide for future fluid intake when you exercise.

Following this practical approach to fluid intake can contribute to well-being. If you're feeling a little more tired or hungry than usual, check to see if you are adequately hydrated. Just having something to drink may be the simplest and fastest solution.

FIBER

Another vital nutrient we've all heard a lot about is fiber. But what is it, exactly, and why is it so important for your health? Dietary fiber is the indigestible parts of fruits, vegetables, beans, nuts, whole grains, and other plant foods. Fiber is what gives celery its crunch, for instance. In your intestines, fiber absorbs water and helps move digestion along; it acts a bit like a broom to sweep out waste. Technically, fiber is a type of carbohydrate, but because it's mostly indigestible, it passes through you and doesn't raise your blood sugar.

The importance of fiber in the diet became clear in the 1970s when Dr. Denis Burkitt and his colleagues published studies on the importance of fiber, based on their work in Africa. Dr. Burkitt hypothesized that certain diseases, such as appendicitis, were more common in Western cultures in part because of lower fiber intake. He noted the impact fiber had on bowel movements and even went as far as to theorize that he could predict the number of hospital visits someone would have based on their type of bowel movements. As it turns out, the effects of fiber are far broader than even Dr. Burkitt suggested.

One of his assumptions about fiber—that it helps prevents colon cancer—is somewhat controversial. Some studies have shown a significant link between a low-fiber diet and colon cancer and also some other types of cancer. On the other hand, Harvard's long-running Nurses' Health Study followed eighty thousand female nurses for nearly two decades and found that fiber was not a significant factor in reducing the risk of colon cancer.

The fiber-cancer link may still be questionable, but there are many other proven reasons to make sure you get enough fiber from your diet. Three of the best reasons are that fiber has been shown to reduce the risk of weight gain, diabetes, and heart disease. Another Harvard study, the long-running Physicians' Health Study, followed forty thousand men for 15 years and found that those with the highest fiber intake had a 40 percent lower risk of heart disease compared to those with the lowest fiber intake. Similar findings were detailed when comparing diets in regard to fiber and sugar intake and the risk of diabetes. A huge study that looked at death from all causes found that those with the highest fiber intake were 22 percent less likely to die over the course of the study than those with the lowest fiber intake.

People who take in more fiber are also better able to control their weight. This works for several reasons. Some research shows that fewer calories are absorbed by the body from high-fiber diets. In addition, a diet high in fiber makes you feel full more quickly and staves off hunger longer as the food takes more time to move through your system. Higher-fiber foods are also less energy dense, meaning they contain fewer calories for the same volume of food. For example, a slice of whole wheat bread has about 70 calories and 2 grams of fiber, while a slice of white bread has about 120 calories and only about 0.6 grams of fiber. Another simple factor may be that fiber foods simply take more chewing. They take longer to eat, which gives your body time to produce the hormones that tell you you're full. Because foods with a lot of fiber take longer to digest, their glucose enters the bloodstream more slowly. This may help avoid insulin surges and let you produce and use insulin more efficiently. Whatever the reason, fiber definitely helps to control weight.

Higher fiber intake can also help lower cholesterol and blood pressure, and it may lower levels of an inflammatory marker called C-reactive protein (CRP). A high level of C-reactive protein in the body can be a sign that the body's process of breakdown and repair has tilted in favor of breakdown. Many studies have shown that consistently high CRP levels are associated with a higher risk of inflammation and of developing heart disease. Increasing your fiber intake is therefore a simple and smart way to keep inflammation down.

So how much fiber do you need? The answer depends on your age and gender. In general, men age 50 or younger need 35 grams of fiber a day; women age 50 or younger need 25 grams a day. Over age 51, the daily requirement drops a bit; men need 30 grams and women need 20 grams daily. Technically, there are two types of fiber: soluble and insoluble fiber. Soluble fiber partially dissolves in water; insoluble fiber resists digestion and doesn't dissolve in water. Both types are important, and both are beneficial, but you don't really need to worry about which type of fiber you're getting. Just aim to consume your daily total from a variety of sources. When you consider that the average American only gets around 15 grams of fiber every day, there is certainly room for improvement. Here are some simple suggestions to help you increase your fiber intake:

- Eat whole grain bread and pasta instead of white bread and semolina pasta. A study of thirty-one thousand Californians in the Adventist Health Study 1 found that those who ate whole wheat bread were a whopping 44 percent less likely to develop coronary artery disease compared to those who ate white bread. This is in line with other studies that show a significant effect from whole grain fiber. Swapping processed white flour for whole grains is a simple dietary change with a huge benefit.

- Eat a higher fiber breakfast cereal. Look for one with at least 4 grams per serving and no added sugar. A lot of tasty choices qualify. You don't have to eat Colon Blow, and it doesn't have to taste like cardboard. Check the label for the fiber content and try some new brands. You may be pleasantly surprised.

- Keep frozen berries handy. They're great for tossing into smoothies and on top of cereal.

- Eat more beans and nuts. Beans are easy to add to soups and stews; nuts can be tossed onto a salad and make a great snack.

- It goes without saying that a good way to add fiber is to add fruits and vegetables, particularly if you eat the peel whenever possible. What's more convenient and tasty than a crispy apple or juicy peach for a snack or dessert? Or some apple slices with a little bit of peanut butter? What about blending in a banana with a smoothie or dipping one into some cocoa powder for a snack? Perhaps add some bell pepper slices, zucchini chunks, or onion onto a grill skewer. Bake a sweet potato instead of a white potato. Keeping cut-up veggies such as carrot sticks in the refrigerator makes it easy to have a fiber-rich snack. Adding veggies to pasta sauce boosts the fiber and adds flavor as well. If you don't feel like munching on these for a snack, think about some popcorn instead.

Adding high-fiber foods to your diet has another valuable benefit: all of those fruits, vegetables, nuts, and so on are rich in other nutrients beyond fiber. You'll be boosting your intake of vital nutrients as you boost your fiber.

Increasing your fiber intake isn't difficult. Find the high-fiber foods that fit your tastes and lifestyle, and make it a priority to eat more of them. Increase your fiber intake slowly over a period of a few weeks. This will give your digestive system time to adjust and avoid problems such as bloating, gas, and diarrhea from adding too much fiber too quickly. Take a look at the table below to get a general idea of the fiber content in some common foods.

FIBER CONTENT OF COMMON FOODS

Food	Amount	Total Fiber, g
Pinto beans	1/2 cup	7.4
Almonds	1/2 cup	6.4
Peanuts	1/2 cup	6.1
Kidney beans	1/2 cup	5.7
Prunes	1/2 cup	5.7
Green peas	1/2 cup	4.4
Apple, with skin	1 medium	4.4
Sweet potato	1 medium	4.0
Blueberries	1 cup	4.0
Oatmeal	1 cup, cooked	4.0
Blackberries	1/2 cup	3.6
Popcorn	3 cups, air popped	3.5
Banana	1 medium	3.1
Baked potato with skin	1 medium	2.9
Broccoli	1/2 cup	2.8
Grapefruit	1 medium	2.9
Kale	1 cup, cooked	2.6
Carrots	1/2 cup	2.6
Corn	1/2 cup	2.0
Whole wheat bread	1 slice	2.0
Strawberries	1/2 cup	1.7
Tomato	1 medium	1.5
White bread	1 slice	0.6
Iceberg lettuce	1/2 cup	0.4

SUPPLEMENTAL VITAMINS, MINERALS, AND ANTIOXIDANTS

Nearly half of all Americans take a daily vitamin/mineral supplement of some kind. The thinking has traditionally been that since most of us could use a little help with our nutritional efforts, taking a daily multivitamin is an easy and convenient way to make up whatever shortages we may have. We've already explored the pitfalls of taking these substances out of their natural context. Unfortunately, the conclusion shared by many health-care providers, has generally been that even if vitamin pills aren't as good as eating vitamin-rich foods, they can't hurt and you have nothing to lose by taking them. This theory has come under heavy fire recently.

MULTIVITAMINS

The standard multivitamin with minerals has been the main beneficiary of this thinking, and yet the data supporting that they are beneficial are very limited. In fact, there is now some evidence that they may actually be harmful.

The Iowa Women's Health Study followed nearly thirty-nine thousand women for 19 years. Not only did they find no benefit from a multivitamin with minerals, but they also found that those who took a daily multi-pill had a 2.4 percent *higher* death rate than those who didn't. This was true even though the multivitamin users generally had a healthier lifestyle. One confounding variable in this study could be estrogen use, but nonetheless, it's a red flag regarding over-reliance on multivitamins. The Iowa study is also significant because it looked at other lifestyle parameters, such as exercise.

Other studies have shown a similar lack of benefit from taking multivitamins. Some scientists have questioned whether the lack of benefit in those other studies is because the vitamin users were generally less healthy, which is why they were taking the pills in the first place. My experience, however, is the opposite. More often than not, my patients who take multivitamins tend to be more health conscious, not less. They eat more whole foods and less junk food, and they generally also take other supplements beyond vitamins and minerals. This surely raises valid questions about the merit of the multivitamin supplements.

A large study published in the *American Journal of Epidemiology* added weight to the argument that multivitamins are of little real value in the prevention of disease. The study followed one hundred eighty thousand people over 11 years and found that multivitamins offered no protection against heart disease or cancer. This is in line with numerous previous studies.

It appears unlikely that a multivitamin is ever going to make an impact on conditions as serious as heart disease or cancer. In fact, there simply isn't enough evidence to prove their merit in any area. Vitamins and supplements are a prime example of the battle between health and wealth. They represent a multibillion-dollar industry.

At this time, I simply can't recommend the use of multivitamins as either a preventive measure or safety net. Studies that cast doubt on their effectiveness *and* their safety continue to be published. It is far wiser to spend your money on healthy foods.

MINERALS

Most people who say they take a daily vitamin pill are actually taking a vitamin pill with minerals. These formulas vary quite a bit but usually contain the minerals calcium, potassium, magnesium, and iron, often in conjunction with a long list of trace minerals, including many that don't even have established recommended daily allowances (RDAs). Because it's rare for anyone to be truly deficient in any of the important minerals—even iron—and even rarer for someone to be deficient in a trace mineral such as vanadium, I don't usually recommend taking these products.

The mineral magnesium, however, is the one mineral supplement that I believe may be helpful. You need magnesium for hundreds of metabolic activities. Magnesium is a key component in the chemical process within your mitochondria that turns glucose into energy. You also need magnesium to build glutathione (your body's most abundant natural antioxidant), to keep your nerves and muscles functioning normally, to keep your heart beating normally, and to build healthy bones.

People who exercise heavily can run low on magnesium, possibly because they eliminate more of it by sweating. If you exercise a lot, raising your magnesium level may improve your endurance and help you recover faster from an intense workout session. People with diabetes or high blood insulin levels are often low on magnesium, possibly because they excrete more of it in their urine. Increasing the magnesium level of someone with diabetes to normal numbers may improve insulin sensitivity and glucose metabolism. We don't know for sure, however, if being low on magnesium makes you more likely to develop type 2 diabetes.

The adult RDA for magnesium is 420 mg for men and 320 mg for women. Many Americans don't meet this daily requirement, mostly because there's little magnesium in processed foods. Good dietary sources of magnesium include nuts, beans, dark green leafy vegetables, whole grains, yogurt, and seafood.

If you're low on magnesium, eating more foods high in this mineral may not raise your levels enough. Your doctor will probably recommend a supplement, usually in the form of magnesium citrate or magnesium threonate. Because too high a dose of magnesium supplements can cause diarrhea and digestive upsets, use them with caution. Begin with a low dose and work up to no more than 600 mg a day. Cut back if you start having bowel problems.

ANTIOXIDANTS

When you drive your car, the engine burns gasoline and converts it to energy to move the vehicle. In the process, the car produces exhaust fumes. In the cells of your body, the many metabolic processes that keep you alive also produce waste products. Some of the waste is in the form of free radicals. Free radicals are atoms or molecules that have an unpaired electron. When an atom or molecule is missing an electron, it becomes unstable and very reactive. It will grab an electron from the nearest atom, even if that means damaging the cell the atom is in. Fortunately, your body has an efficient system of antioxidants—enzymes and other compounds—that shut down free radicals by safely giving them the electrons they need before they can do any harm.

Free radicals can do a lot of damage to your cells, including damaging the DNA in the nucleus. Up to a point, however, free radicals are necessary for normal bodily function. For example, your immune system uses free radicals to kill bacteria. However, when the balance tilts toward free radical predominance, damage to your health can occur. This is where antioxidants come in. They restore the balance, quenching the free radicals and stopping the destructive process.

One way to increase your body's supply of naturally occurring antioxidants is through exercise. Regular resistance exercise help the body's antioxidant defenses become more active. The major source of antioxidants, however, is from your diet. Some vitamins and minerals are antioxidants themselves; others are needed to build antioxidant enzymes. Clearly, having a good diet is beneficial and reduces disease. Foods that are rich in natural antioxidants, such as those from the polyphenol family, are particularly good for health. Foods high in polyphenols include berries, apples, citrus fruits, grapes, and all the colorful vegetables, like carrots and leafy greens.

Will taking supplements of specific antioxidants help? Let's look at the studies on vitamin E, which is a powerful antioxidant, for some answers.

At best, the study results of taking vitamin E are mixed. The results range from showing a benefit to negligible effect to actually causing harm. Part of the problem is that these studies aren't all looking at the same thing. Some looked at vitamin E in isolation; others looked at it in combination with different antioxidants. Others may show different results based on age or gender.

Another significant factor is that in nature, vitamin E is composed of eight different parts. The component researchers focus on, however, is a single part called alpha tocopherol. Alpha tocopherol is the government standard for labeling how much vitamin E is in a supplement; therefore, it's frequently the only part of vitamin E that's included. But isolating just one part of a complex whole and expecting it to do the same as the whole is unrealistic. Alpha tocopherol is the most biologically active part, but that doesn't mean the other seven parts don't play a role. With vitamin E, one example of this is shown in a study where isolated alpha tocopherol supplements didn't protect against Alzheimer's disease, but complete vitamin E from food sources did. Despite this, the most common supplemental form of vitamin E remains alpha tocopherol by itself.

The Physicians' Health Study II is an example of one of many large studies that have looked at antioxidant vitamins. Like many other studies, it found that taking vitamin E supplements had no overall effect on mortality, cardiovascular events, or cancer. Another study showed that taking vitamin E supplements actually increased the risk of prostate cancer by 17 percent.

It's unrealistic to assume that antioxidants alone can prevent such serious conditions. Getting your vitamins, antioxidants, and other nutrients from your food is infinitely superior to getting them from supplements. I used vitamin E as an example because the studies show the problems inherent in looking at the effects of antioxidants, or indeed, any vitamin supplements.

As a physician, I always keep an open mind and look at new data when it comes along. For now, however, there just isn't enough convincing data for me to recommend taking antioxidant supplements. The downside risk *is* real. Beta carotene, a form of vitamin A, was once recommended as an antioxidant supplement to help prevent cancer, among other diseases— until studies in the late 1990s found that taking beta carotene could trigger lung cancer in smokers and former smokers and that it might also lead to prostate cancer.

What about other antioxidants that aren't vitamins, such as resveratrol, a compound found in red wine, chocolate, grapes, and some berries? All too often, when we look more closely at them, these antioxidants don't stand up to the marketing hype. The resveratrol in red wine, for instance, was thought to be the reason having a daily glass seemed to reduce the risk of heart disease. Recent research has shown, however, that resveratrol has no effect one way or the other on your health.

I hold out hope that researchers will find antioxidants that can be taken as supplements and have a positive effect. My gut feeling, however, is that, like vitamin E and resveratrol, their promise will evaporate when enough time for follow-up study has elapsed. When you take something out of its natural form, amplify it, and take it in isolation—without complementary substances that affect everything from its absorption to its function—it is unlikely to have a substantial benefit. In fact, it has the potential for harm.

VITAMIN D

When it comes to vitamins, vitamin D is a special case—the evidence supporting the use of this supplement is much stronger. Vitamin D is unique because it doesn't come from your food. Instead, your body creates it through a complex process that begins when your skin is exposed to sunlight. Because of this difference, the science behind vitamin D supplements is strong and appears to hold significant promise.

Vitamin D has been associated with lower rates of certain cancers, heart disease, high blood pressure, stroke, diabetes, infectious diseases, and even autoimmune diseases such as multiple sclerosis. At a recent meeting of the American Heart Association, material was presented that linked low vitamin D levels with a number of the components of the metabolic syndrome (insulin resistance syndrome), including higher triglycerides, lower good (HDL) cholesterol, higher blood sugars, and higher weight. In a study published in the *Archives of Internal Medicine*, people with the lowest vitamin D levels were twice as likely to die over the nearly eight-year study compared to those with the highest levels of vitamin D.

For years, we've known that certain diseases, such as breast cancer, Crohn's disease, and multiple sclerosis, are more common the farther away you are from the equator. Many researchers believe that people who live at higher latitudes get less exposure to sunshine and have decreased vitamin D levels as a result. It's possible that low vitamin D levels is the underlying cause of these and other diseases.

For most of us today, getting enough sunshine on our skin to produce adequate vitamin D often isn't possible. We don't as a society spend a lot of times outdoors, we wear sunscreen when we do, and many us don't live in places where adequate sun is available during the winter. For instance, if you live north of the line from San Francisco to Washington, DC, from November through February, the sun isn't strong enough for you to make adequate vitamin D, even if you have plenty of sun exposure. In addition, as we get older, our bodies aren't as good at making vitamin D from the sun. The more skin pigmentation you have, the longer it takes to produce vitamin D from the sun exposure. Even having a tan will reduce your production of vitamin D.

Our lack of sun exposure means that we need to get extra vitamin D in other ways. Unlike all the other vitamins, vitamin D isn't found in many foods. Oily fish, egg yolks, butter, and beef liver all contain some; plant foods have virtually none. Vitamin D is added to some foods, including milk, margarine, many breakfast cereals, and some juice brands, but this still isn't enough for the average American to reach adequate blood levels.

The most convenient and certain way of getting enough vitamin D is by taking supplements. In my opinion, based on the science, the current government recommendations for vitamin D intake are too low. The current recommended daily allowance for an adult under age 70 is 600 IU, or 15 micrograms; over age 70, the RDA goes up to 800 IU (20 mcg). When blood levels of vitamin D were measured in studies showing benefit, the levels that were effective for prevention generally couldn't be achieved by following the current government recommendations.

Richard and Susan are two patients who both had low vitamin D levels. They were each taking 800 IU daily in supplemental form, but on their blood tests, they were still significantly below the level associated with benefit. For both, I added an additional 2,000 IU daily. That turned out to be the extra amount they both needed to raise their blood levels. On their next blood tests, they were at the optimal level for vitamin D.

Like Richard and Susan, most people will need to exceed the current recommendations to experience the full benefits of vitamin D. Based on my experience with my patients, supplements are almost always helpful. I use a simple blood test to check the vitamin D levels of my patients. If they are low, as most are, I recommend taking supplements. Some of my patients need 3,000 to 5,000 units daily to get up to a good level, but most do well with around 1,000 units a day.

I also recommend getting some direct sun exposure whenever possible. Just 10 to 15 minutes of sun exposure to the hands and face two or three times a week can give your vitamin D levels a good boost. To give you an insight into just how beneficial sunlight can be, just 20 to 30 minutes of full-body sun exposure to a young person in the summer can produce 20,000 units of vitamin D. You store vitamin D in your body for a long time, so each period of sun exposure puts vitamin D "in the bank" to be used by the body when it's needed.

Obviously, there is a risk of skin cancer from excessive sun exposure, so I'm not advocating we completely stop using sunscreen. I do think, however, that there is a point where the increased vitamin D level from sun exposure and the diseases it prevents outweigh the risk of skin cancer.

Nearly all nonprescription vitamin D supplements contain cholecalciferol, also known as vitamin D3, which is the type your body makes from the sun. Look on the label to be sure you're buying this form and not the less effective form called ergocalciferol, or vitamin D2. The D2 form isn't as potent as D3 and doesn't last as long in the body.

OMEGA-3 FATTY ACIDS

Omega-3 fatty acids are most commonly found in fish and fish oil supplements; they're also found in flaxseeds and flaxseed oil. Dark green leafy vegetables such as kale and collards also contain omega-3 fatty acids, as do nuts, seeds, whole grains, and beans. As we discussed in Chapter 3, omega-3 fatty acids can change the composition of the membrane that encloses every cell in your body. The cell membrane lets water and nutrients into the cell and lets waste products pass out. Oils like omega-3 fatty acids make up a substantial part of the membrane. They make the membrane more responsive to signals and better able to control what goes in and comes out of the cell. That, in turn, makes the cell more responsive to signals and better able to communicate with the cells around it.

Having a high omega-3 content in your cell membranes may help protect you against heart disease, stroke, cancer, arthritis, autoimmune diseases, dementia, depression, and macular degeneration (a common cause of blindness), among other ailments. A good level of omega-3 fatty acids in your body can also help improve your cholesterol profile and protect your memory, and may help stabilize heart rhythms. This might sound too good to be true, but omega-3 fatty acids are being examined against a tough scientific standard—and the results hold up. I believe that eating fish and taking fish oil supplements has the potential to be one of the most beneficial dietary strategies today.

To understand why omega-3 fatty acids are thought to have such rich potential, we need to go back to the two opposing forces in your body. One force promotes inflammatory change and breakdown, and the other fights that breakdown with repair. This battle is being fought in your cells every day. Like any battle, the more soldiers you have on your side the better. Think of the fatty acids in your cell's membrane as the soldiers on the frontline of your health battle. The bad guys are called arachidonic acid (AA), which are a type of omega-6 fatty acid. AA is involved in the production of inflammatory substances and pain in your body. (Actually, you need some omega-6 fatty acids, including AA, for normal body functions. It's when the balance is off that your body becomes inflamed more easily.) The good guys are the omega-3 fatty acids. These have four main components, but the two you need to remember are eicosapentanoic acid (EPA) and decosahexaenoic acid (DHA). The bad guys produce a range of substances that promote inflammation, narrow blood vessels, and encourage blood clotting; the good guys (EPA and DHA) promote the opposite.

Both the bad guys and the good guys compete for the same set of enzymes to get their jobs done. That's where supplementation comes in. If you recruit more omega-3 soldiers to arm your front line through greater intake of omega-3s, then your good army is strengthened and makes up a larger proportion of the cell membrane. When there are more omega-3 fatty acids competing with the bad guys (omega-6s like arachidonic acid) for the enzymes, then the good guys win more often. The result is that you make fewer inflammatory compounds and more protective ones.

In addition, omega-3 fatty acids also seem to play a role in which genes are turned on and which genes are turned off. This is another example of how we can change how our genes work for or against us. Omega-3 fatty acids affect which genes are working in the liver. When you have plenty of omega-3s available, the genes in your liver are shifted toward making and storing less fat there. The end result of this is less insulin resistance and could additionally explain why omega-3 fatty acids are so protective against heart disease, cancer, stroke, dementia, and other serious ailments.

Before exploring how much omega-3 you need and where to get it, it's important to understand that there's a difference between the omega-3 fatty acids in fish oil and those in flaxseeds and flaxseed oil. This difference also holds true for soybean oil, canola oil, and walnut oil, which also have some omega-3 content. The difference is that fish oil has EPA and DHA in ready-to-use form—your body absorbs it right away. The other food items contain alpha linolenic acid (ALA), which needs to be converted in your body to EPA and DHA. The conversion process is slow and inefficient. If you take flaxseed supplements, you won't actually end up with much EPA and DHA from them. This is not to say that the other forms aren't good—just that fish oil is significantly more potent.

While I am always in favor of getting nutrients from whole foods, trying to get all your omega-3 from eating fish may cause another problem. Almost all commonly eaten fish today are contaminated with low levels of mercury, pesticides, and other toxins. Sadly, this is true for both farmed and wild-caught fish. As a result, it seems prudent not to overindulge in fish, especially for children and pregnant women. I'm not saying you shouldn't eat fish. Just the opposite—I think you should aim to eat it two to three times a week. It's just that I don't believe you can consistently get the amount of omega-3 fatty acids you need for the greatest benefit from eating fish alone without also increasing your risk from these other toxins.

There are some types of fish we should probably just avoid, including swordfish, king mackerel, shark, and tilefish, because they have consistently high mercury levels. All fish have some omega-3s, but fatty fish have the most. Good choices include salmon, tilapia, fresh tuna, mahi mahi, trout, red snapper, and sardines. Shellfish and shrimp are also good choices.

If fish contain toxins, does fish oil have them as well? Interestingly, studies have looked for these same toxins in popular brands of fish oil supplements, and the results have been very favorable. Eating fish two or three times each week and increasing your omega-3 intake with fish oil supplements would therefore seem to be the best solution.

On days when you don't eat fish, I recommend supplementing with a minimum of 500 mg of EPA/DHA. Getting extra omega-3s at least three to four times weekly is a reasonable way to be sure your levels stay high. To help with particular health issues, such as depression or high triglycerides, larger amounts may be needed. In such cases, discuss fish oil with a knowledgeable doctor before you try large doses.

When you buy fish oil, check the label for the combined EPA/DHA content, not the total amount of fish oil. For example, if the label says each capsule has 1,200 mg of fish oil, and 220 mg of it is EPA and 150 mg of it is DHA, the total EPA/DHA content would be 370 mg. To get the recommended amount of 500 mg of the two combined, you would have to take two capsules.

To save you the math, many brands now refer to the EPA/DHA combination as total omega-3s. Look for a brand that has all you need in one capsule. Check the label before you buy so you know exactly what you are getting.

Fish oil supplements are best taken with a meal so they will be better absorbed. Ideally, fish oil comes in flavorless capsules, but if you get a fishy aftertaste or fishy burps, or just have an aversion to fish in general, freeze the capsules. Swallow them frozen to avoid these issues.

SECTION 3
EXERCISE

CHAPTER 7
STRENGTH TRAINING

THE BENEFITS OF STRENGTH training have been known for decades to athletes, trainers, and people like the "godfather of fitness," Jack LaLanne. The medical community has taken much longer to catch on. Plenty of studies show that muscular strength, independent of aerobic fitness (your ability to transport and utilize oxygen), is linked to reduced rates of heart disease, diabetes, Alzheimer's disease, insulin resistance, and the full-blown metabolic syndrome. In a 2011 study in the *Journal of Clinical Endocrinology & Metabolism* of over thirteen thousand people, an almost linear relationship was found between adding muscle through strength training and reducing insulin resistance. The researchers found that for each 10 percent increase in skeletal muscle, there was an 11 percent reduction in insulin resistance. Interestingly, the link was stronger among people who didn't have diabetes than those who already did have diabetes. The reasons for this are complex, but the overall conclusion—that having more or better muscle improves insulin efficiency—is easy to grasp. Muscular strength is also independently linked to reduced death rates from *all* causes, including cancer, even after adjusting for aerobic fitness.

The effects of strength training are independent of aerobic fitness. Training your muscles provides additional benefits beyond strength alone—being strong but not aerobically fit was still protective.

However, building strength isn't as simple as just using the machines at the gym. Good muscular strength—the kind that can best lower your weight, risk of disease, and premature death—requires a workout program that incorporates frequent and appropriate changes, varies in the specifics of what you do, and takes you along a proper progression for optimal results.

The importance of this progression is well illustrated in the GREAT2DO trial, an important study published in 2013. The study was one of the biggest to look at the benefits of progressive strength training compared to a program that included strength training but didn't make the workout more difficult over time. The researchers compared participants who worked out three times a week and did progressive strength training (they gradually increased the amount of weight they lifted over the course of a year) to participants who also worked out three times a week but didn't increase the amount of weight they lifted. Specifically, the researchers looked at the effect on insulin resistance and average blood sugar of progressive resistance training. What they found was eye-opening. Participants in the progressive group who gained muscle had significant reductions in insulin resistance and average blood sugar compared to those who worked out but didn't make their routine more difficult over time. I want to emphasize that the people who benefited the most were compared to others who were *also* spending the same amount of time exercising. In addition, the positive changes were independent of body weight. Even the people who were overweight saw benefits when they went to progressive training.

The very basic progressive strength-training program used in the GREAT2DO trial provided remarkable benefits. But what if you varied the exercise choices, order, speed, and techniques? Not only would the program be a lot more interesting and fun to stick with, but it also would give you even better results. And that's exactly what the YOU+ program does. The YOU+ techniques lead to definite improvements in muscle tone, muscle strength, and weight loss—and also in insulin efficiency. With a properly sequenced program of progressive strength training, you can avoid being one of the people I often see at the gym doing the usual uninspired, unchallenging routines.

When you add aerobic fitness to strength training, the benefits are even greater. I believe this is true in part because of the way both forms of exercise improve insulin efficiency and cause an additive reduction in insulin resistance, more than would be expected from either type of exercise alone. Even if you're not insulin resistant, keeping your insulin levels as low as possible will help you reach your health and fitness goals.

In one study of more than eight thousand men ranging in age from 20 to 75, the combination of being both strong and fit led to a marked reduction in the risk of developing the metabolic syndrome. The participants who were both strong and fit, even if they were overweight, were at least 62 percent less likely to have the metabolic syndrome. As these and many other studies show, working out clearly has powerful health benefits for men and women at any age.

But what you do during your workout and how you do it makes a difference. The YOU+ method helps you make the most of your exercise while taking this principle to the next level. By using the YOU+ app or website, you will learn, through step-by-step workouts and other tools, how to incorporate strength training and aerobic fitness using advanced techniques that go beyond those already proven to be successful.

STRENGTH TRAINING AND YOUR WEIGHT

Strength training provides many benefits beyond disease prevention. Among other things, it will also help you achieve your desired weight. In simple terms, working out burns more calories than sitting still does, so you would expect to lose some weight just from the increased activity. But strength training seems to have a greater effect on weight loss than you would expect just from burning more calories. It's not just a matter of calories in versus calories burned. Based on my extensive personal experience in the gym and my experience working with my patients, I believe that the improved insulin efficiency that comes from strength training has a significant impact on losing weight and keeping it off. That's why the YOU+ program helps with weight loss beyond just calories burned.

It gets better.

Experts disagree about exactly how many calories a pound of muscle burns relative to a pound of body fat. They all agree, however, that muscle is more metabolically active than fat, which means that the more muscles you have, the more calories you burn just by being alive. I think the more practical way to look at it is not by how many calories are burned per pound of muscle, but rather by what happens to your metabolic rate and fat burning with a strength-training program. This is the best way to see what happens to your total calorie burn, rather than just looking at the calorie furnace.

From this perspective, one study showed that a strength-training program that put on three pounds of muscle and took off four pounds of fat increased the subjects' metabolic rate by about 7 percent. That's the equivalent to burning an extra 120 calories per day, every day. While this may not sound like much, burning just 120 extra calories a day from the effects of strength training can have a significant cumulative effect. One pound of fat is the equivalent of 3,500 calories. Every time you accumulate 3,500 more calories than you need, you gain a pound. Every time you burn 3,500 more calories than you take in, you lose a pound. Over the course of a year, using 120 calories more every day means you would lose more than 12 pounds. That's weight you lose because your excess fat is being used up by the muscles you gained by strength training.

Over the course of a year of strength training, you'll be stronger, even though you weigh less. You would have to spend a *lot* of time on a treadmill to get the same results you get from strength training. If one of your fitness goals is weight management, then strength training is the way to go.

USE IT OR LOSE IT

Strength training will improve your quality of life. To live your life actively and enjoyably, you need to be able to participate in all of the activities of your daily life without strain. Studies show that people who strength train are more active in the other areas of their life than people who don't strength train. In other words, they have the capacity to live their life more fully. My experience with patients has shown that in activities ranging from travel to pastimes to sex, those who work out participate in activities more often than those who don't. Even in everyday activities— such as climbing onto the kitchen counter to get something from a high shelf, lifting the kids or grandkids, or just carrying your packages a few blocks in the city without having to hail a cab—strength matters. In the long term, people who strength train are significantly less likely to end up in a nursing home than those who don't.

The undeniable truth about strength is that if you don't use it, you *will* lose it. The average sedentary person loses about one-third of a pound of muscle every year after the age of 35.

After losing that much muscle yearly for a decade, you will have lost just over 3 pounds of muscle, and that number will keep growing over time unless you do something about it. With less muscle, you burn fewer calories and gain weight. That's where middle-aged weight gain comes from.

It doesn't have to be that way, as the example I gave above shows. Three pounds of muscle gained from a strength program can save 12 pounds a year in weight gain. Take that one step further. Those 3 pounds are equivalent to the amount of muscle lost by a sedentary person every ten years after the age of 35. I have often heard patients who don't engage in any strength training tell me that they are gaining weight even though they are doing nothing differently. That's the point—once you reach the age where muscle loss inevitably begins, doing nothing differently automatically means weight gain. Bottom line: you will lose muscle and gain weight unless you reverse that process through strength training.

In addition to losing muscle mass as we age, the quality of the muscle that's left worsens. This means that you have less strength per pound of muscle you retain. Think of your muscles as a jar of hot chili powder. One tablespoon when you first open the jar has a lot more kick to it than one tablespoon after a year in the cabinet. The same is true for the strength of your muscles.

Muscle power also decreases as we age. Muscle power is, in simple terms, being able to generate a lot of force quickly. Many authorities feel that the loss of muscle power is the most important factor in the decreasing ability to do things over time. This may seem like an academic distinction, but it's important when considering how to put together a training program.

These changes can create a triple whammy: you have less muscle, the muscle you do have isn't as good, *and* it's less powerful. This all sounds pretty discouraging, but there is good news.

You can prevent most of this from ever happening to you. And if much of it has already happened to you, you can dramatically reverse the decline. This goes for everything about your muscles: muscle mass, strength, quality, and power.

We've known this to be true ever since the 1980s. An important study back then showed that 12 weeks of strength training could create substantial improvement in muscle mass and strength even though the participants in the study ranged in age from 60 to 72 years old. Other studies since then have shown strength gains beyond what would be expected from increased muscle mass alone, which indicates that training also improves muscle quality. Improvements in muscle power have also been repeatedly documented. There are even many studies demonstrating that people in their 90s have dramatic responses to weight training. So whatever your age, you are definitely never too old to benefit from strength training!

The debate in the academic world now centers on the mechanism of *how* this happens, rather than *if* it happens. This debate is important from the YOU+ perspective because it sheds light on the best, most efficient, and safest way to train to get the results you want.

Sadly, many health professionals don't fully understand the advantages of strength training or who can benefit from it. The father of one of my daughter's friends, for example, was recently advised not to weight train because of mild hypertension. The reality is that the long-term effect of weight training can help lower high blood pressure. It can even help people who have congestive heart failure.

Even well-informed health professionals who recognize the benefits of weight training don't typically know what to recommend to their patients. If your physician or other health-care professional has recommended the YOU+ program, you can be assured that he or she is on the cutting edge.

Though the improvement in your well-being from strength training can be substantial, I'm not saying that older folks will be able to match teenagers. After all, there aren't too many 80-year-old professional athletes or Olympians. There are, however, a lot of Senior Olympians who easily outdo younger people. A patient once told me about his friend, who wanted to start weight training to help him qualify for the Senior Olympics. His physician advised against it, believing that weight training was inadvisable in general for anyone his age. This gentleman ignored the advice and began weight training anyway. He continued to improve his strength and skills and did in fact participate in the Senior Olympics. He did very well, but unfortunately, by then, his doctor had died from a heart attack and wasn't alive to see it.

WHERE TO TRAIN

OK, it's pretty obvious that you need strength training in your exercise regimen. The only question left in your mind now is where should you work out. You basically have two choices: at home or at a gym. Working out at home has some advantages, including the time saved by not having to travel to and from the gym, privacy, and not having to wait for access to equipment. Home gym equipment is now quite good, but you could just as easily buy an inexpensive set of free weights (dumbbells or barbells) and get the same benefits. If you are highly self-motivated or have financial or time limitations, then working out in your home gym might be the best choice for you. An effective program can be designed for home workouts. The YOU+ app and website includes a home program that will teach you the proper strength-training regimen using only a set of dumbbells and an exercise ball.

If it's feasible, however, joining your local gym is preferable. Working out in a well-equipped gym offers a number of important benefits that you will always miss out on in a home gym environment. The main advantage is that a gym will have a wide range of equipment for both strength work and aerobic training. This not only provides the variety needed to give you the full benefits of exercise, but it also goes a long way in preventing boredom. Having other people around can also be helpful. The gym has the right environment and energy level to help you meet your personal goals—other people in the gym tend to be supportive and encouraging. In fact, you'll probably make some workout friends if you're the sociable sort.

Many people find it helpful to have a dedicated place to go for the specific purpose of working out—the many distractions at home can influence even the best of intentions. There's also the cost. Many people assume that joining a gym will be more expensive than setting up a home gym, but the reality can be quite different. You can belong to many gyms for quite some time for what you would spend on a good home exercise system—these can cost several thousand dollars. Basic dumbbells and an exercise ball, are very inexpensive, but even a simple weight setup takes up space that you might not have in your home.

If you are going to invest in one piece of home equipment, I would suggest that you get something for your cardiovascular work. You can do aerobic work on an exercise bike, treadmill, or elliptical trainer at home while watching a movie or TV. Do the weight work at the gym if you can.

FINDING THE RIGHT GYM

If you're going to join a gym, finding the right one can make a big difference in your ultimate success. It has to be a place where you will actually go, so you need feel comfortable there. The most important factor is probably location. If the gym isn't convenient for you, you simply won't go as often as you need to—and you may eventually stop going at all. Convenience has a lot to do with where you will be traveling from when you go to work out. Will it be from home, from work, or maybe from someplace where you often are, such as your child's school? Finding a gym near this destination will make it easier to go. Your workplace might have a gym that would be convenient for you (and maybe even free or reduced rate). If a gym that's part of a chain is near you, it may offer access to all of its other locations—even the ones in other parts of town, which can make working out even more convenient.

I think it's very important to visit a gym you're thinking of joining before you make a commitment. Every gym, even the chains, has a different feel or personality, and you can sense this by visiting. Look at the age range and gender of the folks who are working out there. Are they primarily bodybuilders, moms with kids, older adults, or a good mix of everybody? You need to feel that you will be comfortable in whatever mix of patrons the gym has. Some women feel most comfortable with a women-only gym.

Check out how crowded the gym is by visiting at a time when you're most likely to be there. You don't want to be constantly waiting for the piece of equipment or find yourself closed out of an exercise class. A gym looks very different at 10:00 in the morning versus 6:00 in the evening. Make sure the gym's hours suit your needs. This is especially important if you plan to work out in the early morning or late at night. Many, but not all, gyms are now open 24 hours a day, 7 days a week. Some also offer child care while you work out—be sure to check out the available hours and space if you plan to use this service.

Also check out the staff and facilities. Are the people who work there friendly and helpful? Is the facility clean and well maintained? The locker rooms should be clean, and the equipment should be in good working order. Check to see if the machines are sturdy and move smoothly, without excessive noise. You don't want to see any frayed cables or rusty dumbbells. You also need to see if the gym has a good range of high-quality equipment that's appropriate for the workouts you're planning. In addition to cardio equipment, free weights, and weight machines, does the gym offer any classes, such as aerobics, spinning, or yoga? You might be interested in water exercises or racquetball. Does the gym have a well-maintained pool? What are the racquetball courts like?

Once you find a place that might work for you, give it a trial run. Don't be afraid to ask for a free pass. Many gyms will give you one if they know you are interested in joining and not just seeking a free workout. If you decide to join the gym, don't feel pressured into signing anything. Find out how long the contract is for and if it renews automatically, which could mean that your membership is renewed even if you don't want to. Find out if classes are extra, and try to get a month-to-month, pay-as-you-go plan if possible. The fees and the length of the contract may be negotiable, particularly up-front fees. Find out about the cancellation policy in case your situation changes. This will protect you from any surprises later on. All in all, signing up should be a painless process. If it isn't, you should probably look somewhere else. The cost of gym membership will depend on where you live and how fancy you want your gym to be, but around $30 to $60 a month would be reasonable.

WHAT ABOUT A TRAINER?

Whether you work out at home or at the gym, it's always wise to have at least one session with a personal trainer to ensure that you learn the proper form and technique for using the weights and exercise machines that are a central part of the YOU+

program. This is vital to success. Not long ago, I was in the gym with a couple of friends. We all stopped to marvel at one man who was making a lot of noise while doing a particular exercise. Unfortunately for him, his technique and form were all wrong. He thought he was getting fit, but he was actually damaging his body. Chances are he would soon have been in his doctor's office, complaining of pain. That bad experience would then keep him from going back to the gym—all because he didn't know the correct technique and form in the first place.

Even slightly incorrect form can eventually lead to an injury, but learning proper form can prevent this. This should be one of the primary roles of the trainer you work with. You don't need someone to give you advice that strays from the fundamentals discussed in this book and explained in the YOU+ app and website. You also don't need someone to sell you supplements. You need someone to teach you how to perform the exercises correctly, and for that, a good trainer can be indispensable. A good trainer will also help you shape and tailor your workouts to meet your goals and abilities, while minimizing your risk of injury.

Because I place a high value on having at least one session with a trainer, choosing the right trainer is important. A reasonable place to start is the trainer's certification. Huge disparities in this area make certification a bit hard to understand. Some certifications come from a lot of serious course work and a comprehensive written exam. In fact, some colleges now offer bachelor's degree programs in personal training. Then there are the "certifications" that can be purchased just by taking a short online course. Some people who call themselves trainers have no certification at all. They may have a lot of experience in the gym, but you have no way of knowing for sure if they really know what they're talking about.

Ideally, the process of certification will be regulated someday. In the meantime, look for a trainer who has certification from one of the following professional associations:

- American Council on Exercise (ACE)

- American College of Sports Medicine (ACSM)

- International Sports Sciences Association (ISSA)

- National Academy of Sports Medicine (NASM)

- National Strength and Conditioning Association (NSCA)

- National Federation of Professional Trainers (NFPT)

- National Council on Strength & Fitness (NCSF)

The person you hire definitely needs to be somebody you like and are comfortable with. This is particularly true if you're looking for more than one session. Even one hour can be useless if you don't like or trust the person. You don't have to work out together the first time you meet, and I advise you not to. An initial brief meeting to assess whether this is the person you should hire is essential. A good trainer should be a good listener and be able to accurately assess your current level of fitness. Nothing is more demotivating than starting out too hard and being so sore the next day that you never want to go back. During your session, the trainer should be paying attention only to you, not chatting with other members or doing his or her own workout along with you. Ask about basic logistic issues. Can the trainer work with your schedule? What about being charged if you have to cancel? Does he or she have liability insurance? Ask for personal references. If the trainer is hesitant about this or if you're not happy with his or her certification, move on to the next person on your shortlist.

As with gym memberships, a trainer's fee will vary depending on where you live. Expect to pay around $50 an hour in most places. Some gyms may offer you a free session with a trainer to get you started after you join. Be sure to ask about this.

You may find that you really like working out with a trainer; but for many, expense becomes an issue over time. Once you've learned about the correct techniques and form from your trainer, I strongly recommend that you consider finding a good workout partner instead. If you feel you're having trouble with your form, however, or you're having difficulty with a new piece of exercise equipment, a session with a trainer might be a good idea.

For me personally, having a workout partner has made a huge difference. Having a training partner isn't for everyone, but it can be the key to the consistency needed for success. A good partner will keep you focused and motivated and make it easier to exercise. There are days when I just wouldn't have gone to the gym if I didn't have someone there waiting for me. There are days when, even though I am there, my time would have been essentially wasted if I didn't have someone to help me focus my efforts in the right direction.

Perhaps the biggest advantage in having a workout partner is that it makes working out a lot more fun. Having someone you can laugh with, kid around with, or sometimes even compete with helps to keep the gym fresh and interesting. Fun in the gym may sound like an oxymoron to many, but with the right training partner—perhaps a friend or equally committed work colleague—your workout really can be fun. You can transform it from something that's a chore into something you actually look forward to.

CHAPTER 8
THE YOU+ STRENGTH-TRAINING PLAN

W HAT'S THE BEST WAY to begin your strength-training plan? You may be tempted to dive right into a training regimen, but let's stop and think about that first. A little patience now will go a long way toward your future success.

As we think about how to get you started in the best way, let's look at where you are now. Perhaps you're already working out but aren't seeing the results you want. Or maybe you've never really been much of an exerciser and don't know where to begin. Or maybe you've worked out in the past, but you gave up out of boredom and lack of progress. You'd like a proven way to get back to fitness with better results.

Regardless of which scenario best describes you, I believe you should start by looking at your time in the gym as a series of progressive steps. Once you have successfully completed each of two brief initial stages, you will be experienced enough in the gym to follow a general set of principles for the long haul.

The principles I'll lay out for you here, and in the YOU+ app and website, maximize your fight against higher-than-needed insulin levels. You'll have greater insulin efficiency—and that will pay off not just in the gym but also in every other aspect of your health—from weight control to disease prevention.

In the YOU+ program, you'll start by using the YOU+ app or website to answer a series of questions about your lifestyle. Depending on your responses, the appropriate starting point for you will be determined. Even if you're already a regular at the gym, it's important to answer the questions and get feedback customized just for you.

If you're new to working out, the YOU+ program moves you through three stages. The first stage lasts two weeks, and the second lasts four weeks. The third stage lasts the rest of your life, giving you strength and vitality that applies to everything you do.

STAGE ONE

Stage One of the YOU+ program is a whole-body workout done on exercise machines only, if at all possible. I'm not an advocate of a machine-only approach, and I don't think everyone needs to work out only in a gym, but it's important to start this way if you can. As your fitness level advances, you'll do less on the machines and more with free weights; if you work out at home, you'll be able to get more from your own exercise equipment. For now, as you get started, machine-only work in a gym helps you learn proper form for working each muscle group. It also reduces your risk of injury. You don't have to worry about balance and coordination because the machine will guide you through the range of motion and help you learn the proper form.

If you can't arrange to do Stage One in a well-equipped gym, it's still perfectly possible to do it using your home equipment. Don't let gym access stand in the way of changing your life.

COMPOUND AND SINGLE-JOINT EXERCISES

In Stage One, we focus on compound exercises to a greater extent than single-joint exercises. Compound exercises are exercises that use more than one joint on the same side of the body at the same time. An example would be using the leg press machine. In this exercise, you're seated and you put both feet, about shoulder-width apart, onto a metal plate holding the weights (whatever amount you feel is right for you). To begin the exercise, you lower the weight by pulling your knees in closer to your chest. You then complete the exercise by pushing the plate away from you until your legs are almost straight.

This is a compound exercise because two joints—your hips and knees—are involved in the motion. Compound exercises are efficient because you work a greater amount of muscle at one time. Studies have shown improvement in many parameters, such as strength and hormone levels, when compound exercises are at the core of a strength-training program.

Single-joint exercises are also part of Stage One. Single-joint exercises, as the name suggests, use only a single joint, such as your knee, elbow, or shoulder. The biceps curl machine is a good example of a single-joint exercise. To do a biceps curl, grasp the handles of the machine, keeping your elbows on the pad. Starting with your arms nearly straight out, curl the weight by moving your palms up toward your shoulders. Only your elbows move, so this is a single-joint exercise.

All of the exercises I discuss here, plus many more, are described and illustrated with how-to videos on the YOU+ app and website. If you're not sure about how to do an exercise, please take a look at it on the app or website first—good form will help you get the most from the exercise and avoid injury.

MIND–MUSCLE CONNECTION

Stage One helps you develop an enhanced connection between your mind and your muscles. This is important for improving your muscle quality. Over time, some of the nerve connections to your muscles deteriorate. With less nerve input, muscle quality fades. Working the muscle restores the nerve pathways and improves muscle quality.

The best results are achieved when you are really able to focus in on the "feel" of the muscle being worked. Being able to isolate the muscle this way takes some time—I wouldn't expect you to master it in Stage One. Because the exercise machines lock you into the correct motion, however, you will begin to mentally connect to the feeling of the muscle working correctly.

STRENGTH TRAINING BASICS

Start your strength training by doing seven exercises that cover your body's major muscle groups. You should always warm up for around five minutes before you start lifting weights. This can best be achieved by some sort of aerobic (cardio) activity, such as a short ride on an exercise bike or a walk on the treadmill. Warming up with aerobics is essential, regardless of how experienced you are in the gym.

WOMEN AND STRENGTH TRAINING

During Stage One, men will do weight training three times a week, and women will do weight training twice a week. I suggest only two sessions a week for women because studies show that women do not recover from resistance training as quickly as men do. They need more recovery time between workouts to avoid overtraining. The greatest benefit for women appears to come when working each muscle group no more than twice a week.

Too frequently, women are discouraged from lifting weights. They're told, or they believe, that weight training will create an overly muscular, unfeminine physique. This is simply not true. This myth has been perpetuated by images of heavily muscled female bodybuilders who use steroid drugs. Instead, women who work out with weights achieve a fit and toned look that can't be accomplished with aerobic exercise alone.

Women who follow the YOU+ program achieve both their desired weight and strong, toned bodies. And they get an additional benefit: stronger bones. A number of studies have shown that improvements in bone density, which protects against osteoporosis, are directly tied to the amount of weight lifted. Women who lift weights get stronger bones, not bigger muscles.

MUSCLE RECOVERY

Often when people start strength training, they think more is better. They'll work out in the gym more often than they should. Don't do it!

Although you work your muscles in the gym, the development of your muscles occurs outside of the gym, during your recovery period. That's when your body repairs and rebuilds the muscle fibers that are broken down by progressive exercise, including weight training. The repair process creates stronger muscles. Your workout starts the muscle-building process; your recovery period consolidates it.

The recovery period for a muscle is at least 48 hours, so you should never work the same muscle two days in a row. Rest and recovery are as important for muscle growth as your workout itself. If you overtrain and don't allow adequate time for muscle recovery, you'll experience a setback with your goals. You'll feel fatigued by your workout instead of energized; you might also injure yourself.

If you're overtraining, you'll have muscle soreness lasting beyond a day or two, persistent fatigue, elevated resting heart rate, irritability, lack of motivation or feeling stale, and diminishing performance. The easiest way to avoid this situation is to ensure that you allow enough recovery time and eat adequate protein (see Chapter 5 for more on diet).

YOUR STAGE ONE ROUTINE

The seven exercises in Stage One work your chest, back, shoulders, biceps, triceps, calves, and legs. For each exercise, you will use a different weight machine. All the machines you need for the Stage One exercises are standard equipment and can be found at almost any gym. If your gym doesn't have some of the suggested equipment, check the YOU+ app or website to find a suitable substitute—use the video to learn how to do the exercise. If you're working out at home, most of the exercises utilize dumbbells, while some are body weight exercises.

In training terminology, a certain number of repetitions (reps) makes up one set of an exercise. A set usually consists of 10 to 15 reps.

Which Gym Machine?

Body Part	Exercise
Chest	Chest press machine
Back	Lat row machine or lat pulldown
Legs	Leg press machine
Biceps	Machine curl
Triceps	Triceps dip machine
Calves	Standing calf raise
Shoulders	Shoulder press machine

Which Home Exercises?

Body Part	Exercise
Chest	Push-up or flat dumbbell press *(women)*
Back	One-arm dumbbell row
Legs	Standing front lunge
Biceps	Dumbbell curl
Triceps	One-arm overhead triceps extension
Calves	One-legged calf raise
Shoulders	Y shoulder press

Complete these exercises in a circuit. In other words, do one set of an exercise, then move on to the next exercise, and so on until you have completed all seven exercises. Rest for one to two minutes between each set. Once you've completed all seven, go back to the beginning and go through the exercises for a second time.

For the first time through, or the first set of each exercise, do 15 repetitions with a weight that is about half the weight that you think you could lift once in that exercise (I'll discuss this more below). The last couple of repetitions should be a bit of an effort, but you shouldn't reach the point where you're unable to do any more than 15—if that happens, you're using too much weight. At the end of the first set of each exercise, you should feel that you could have done a couple more reps with intense effort.

For the second time through, or the second set of each exercise, use more weight than you did the first time. The goal is to reach a point of good effort at 12 repetitions instead of at 15 repetitions as you did the first time through.

"Good effort" means that you really had to concentrate and push yourself to get through those last couple of repetitions on the second set. At my gym, I see people reading a book or talking to a friend while doing this type of exercise routine. *Nothing* will be gained at that level of effort. If you are going to commit to going to the gym, then make it count and make it worth your time. Focus on the exercises and push yourself a bit.

The exception to the 15/12 repetition scheme is for calf and leg exercises, where you should maintain 15 reps for each set.

Use heavier weights for the second set, which will consequently require more effort. Another exception is that women will do only one set of calf exercises.

STARTING WEIGHTS

The biggest challenge most people face when starting their strength training is gauging the correct starting weight. If you have an orientation session with a trainer, you can use that time to get feedback on what your starting weight should be. You can also always make adjustments based on what your experience is once you start working out. In general, you want to be lifting weights heavy enough to make those last few reps really challenging, but not so heavy that you can't maintain good form while completing them.

The purpose is to make it count. If your weights are too light, your workout will be too easy—you're wasting your time. Too heavy, and your workout will be too hard to complete well. You could injure yourself or become too sore, which will discourage you from sticking with it. Toward the end of the second week of Stage One, you'll probably find that your strength is increasing. Adjust the weights you use accordingly.

EXERCISE ORDER

The order of the exercises is important. You should work the big muscle groups (chest, back, legs) before the small ones (shoulders, biceps, triceps, calves). The small muscle groups assist the big muscle groups in their movement. The biceps, for instance, are involved in back movements, and the triceps and shoulders are involved in chest movements. If you work the small muscles first during Stage One, they will be fatigued by the time you get to the big muscles, and they won't be able to handle what they are required to do. The big muscles won't get the workout they need. If you work your biceps before your back, for instance, the biceps will tire before the back does. The back won't get the necessary workout.

Every major muscle is paired with another muscle that is designed to do the opposite motion. For instance, your biceps muscle at the front of your upper arm flexes your arm; the triceps at the back of your upper arm extends it. In these muscle pairs, when one muscle contracts, the other must relax. As you get started with resistance exercise, take advantage of this pairing and order the exercises based on this concept.

The available pairings in the seven exercises outlined in the chart above would be chest-back and biceps-triceps. This means that you should always work these two groups one after the other. Do your back immediately after your chest. Do your triceps immediately after your biceps, or vice versa. As long as you work these pairs together, you can order your circuit in any way you like. For example, you could do chest, back, legs, biceps, triceps, calves, and then shoulders, or you could do back, chest, triceps, biceps, legs, shoulders, and then calves.

The YOU+ app and website provide illustrated workouts to follow and insights to and demonstrations of proper form and technique for resistance training based on your responses to a series of questions. If you aren't sure about the correct form for an exercise, or if you're looking for new exercises to try, YOU+ has answers.

The charts below give examples of a Stage One workout using machines in a gym or in a home setting. The workout starts with the large chest and back muscles and moves on to the legs and then to the biceps/triceps combination, then calves, and ends with the shoulders. The exercises are simple and basic—they're meant to get you started in a positive way. Follow this type of workout for the two weeks of Stage One.

STAGE ONE SAMPLE WORKOUT IN THE GYM

Body Part	Exercise/Machine	1st set	2nd set
Chest	Chest press machine	15 reps	12 reps
Back	Lat row machine or lat pulldown	15 reps	12 reps
Legs	Leg press machine	15 reps	15 reps
Biceps	Machine curl	15 reps	12 reps
Triceps	Triceps dip machine	15 reps	12 reps
Calves	Standing calf raise *only 1 set for women*	15 reps	15 reps
Shoulders	Shoulder press machine	15 reps	12 reps

STAGE ONE SAMPLE WORKOUT AT HOME

Body Part	Exercise/Machine	1st set	2nd set
Chest	Push-up or flat dumbbell press	15 reps	12 reps
Back	One-arm dumbbell	15 reps	12 reps
Legs	Standing front lunge	15 reps	15 reps
Biceps	Dumbbell curl	15 reps	12 reps
Triceps	One-arm overhead triceps extensions	15 reps	12 reps
Calves	One-legged calf raise *only 1 set for women*	15 reps	15 reps
Shoulders	Y shoulder press	15 reps	12 reps

STAGE TWO

During the four weeks of Stage Two, you'll add some free-weight exercises and a second exercise per body part. Now that we're adding more exercises, we need to think of the muscle groups as being in two parts and work them in different workouts to keep from overdoing it or making the workout too long.

Both women and men will work out three times a week. The recovery time issue still holds true for women, but because you are now working different areas across different sessions, no body part will be worked more than twice a week. You'll still have adequate recovery time for each muscle group.

THE BASICS

In Stage Two, we divide the muscles of the body into two working groups:

- **Group 1:** chest, shoulders, and triceps
- **Group 2:** legs, calves, back, and biceps

This approach groups the muscles that are opposite each other into different workout days. The principle of working the large muscles before the small ones still applies. In Stage Two, you will alternate which muscle group you use each workout. In other words, the first workout of the week will be group 1, the second will be group 2, and the third will be back to group 1. You start the next week with group 2, and so on.

If your schedule calls for it, you can now work out two days in a row instead of taking a day or more off in between. Because you're using opposite muscles in each workout, you will be working muscles the next day that weren't used the day before. So, you're still going to have more than the 48 hours of recovery time before you get to each muscle group again.

One caveat: I don't recommend doing resistance exercise more than two days in a row, even if you have recovery time later. Although different muscles would be worked on the different consecutive days, I have found that the body still needs that third day off to maintain the best level of fitness.

For this and any stage of resistance exercise, focus on form is paramount. Concentrate on doing the exercises correctly— which means you're also doing them safely. By now, you should be feeling more comfortable with doing the exercises; you shouldn't have to rely on the exercise machines as much to guide you through the range of motion. In this stage, you will also be working with free weights (barbells and dumbbells). I suggest staying with the gym throughout the four weeks of Stage Two so you can gain more experience with free weights before working out at home on your own. If that's not possible, working out in your home gym is fine.

In Stage Two, you'll begin to notice even greater gains in your strength and muscle quality. Now it's time to move toward working with both the exercise machines and free weights. For each body part, choose one machine exercise and one free-weight exercise The movement toward free weights is important because free weights have a significant advantage over machines. With a machine, you are guided through the exercise, which ensures that your technique and form are correct and consistent. But once you've mastered the correct technique and form, you can start to step away from the machines. Free weights generally produce better results because your body must control the weight and keep it balanced in a way that doesn't happen with the machines. Using free weight means that smaller accessory muscles are also engaged to move the weight through the range of motion of the exercise. To do this, you use nerves that sense where your body parts are in space, without having to look—technically, this is called "proprioception." Making these nerves work to keep the movement in balance is great for maintaining the quality of the connection between your brain and your muscles and improving your coordination and balance.

Free weights are an important component of whole body fitness. They pay off in your day-to-day activities by improving your ability to do things like climb stairs, which requires not only strength but also coordination and balance. And they also play a role in improving sports performance. Another good reason to start adding free weights to your workouts? They let you vary your exercise routine more. You don't get bored with the same old machines, and you get to learn new exercises that use your muscles in different ways.

YOUR STAGE TWO ROUTINE

In Stage Two, you train parts of your body on separate days, alternating between group 1 (chest, shoulders, and triceps) and group 2 (legs, calves, back, and biceps).

When you're working your upper body, use a machine for one exercise and free weights for the other exercise. For your lower body, you can continue to perform both exercises on a machine at this time.

Complete four total sets for each body part. Do this by completing two sets of one exercise and then two sets of the other. The exception to this is your calves, which need only three sets of one exercise for men and two sets of one exercise for women.

Again, the main challenge is selecting the correct starting weight. By now, you know your own capabilities, so this should not be as tricky as Stage One. For your upper body, the first set of each exercise should be a weight about half of what you could lift once for that exercise. Complete 15 repetitions using that weight, just as in Stage One. The second set should be at a weight you can do 10 times, where the ninth and tenth repetitions take quite a bit of effort. Adjust the weight based on how easy or hard each exercise feels. If you can't get to 10 repetitions in your second set, decrease the weight. If you can easily do 10, increase the weight. Adjust the weights, not the number of reps.

Rest for around 90 seconds to 2 minutes between sets.

For your legs and calves, maintain 15 reps for both sets of an exercise (three for men on calves), but after the first set, increase the weight. You should still be able to complete the full 15 reps, but the last few should be a significant effort.

EXERCISE ORDER

The big difference between Stage Two and Stage One is that now, you'll be completing consecutive sets on the same body part, instead of switching body parts after each set. For example, in Stage One, you completed one set of chest exercises and moved on to a different body part. In Stage Two, you'll complete all of your chest exercises consecutively.

During this stage, you'll be doing two exercises for each body part (except your calves, for which you do one exercise): one using the weight machine and one using free weights. Only when you finish working one body part completely do you move on to the next, repeating the process of four sets for each body part in the group.

This may sound like a lot more to do, but, for group one muscles, it's actually two fewer sets than you did in Stage One. The emphasis has been shifted so you can continue to gain further advantage from your time in the gym. The YOU+ app and website have level planners to illustrate what your individualized workout progression should be.

To help you get started on your Stage Two workouts, use the sample exercises in the chart.

STAGE TWO SAMPLE WORKOUT IN THE GYM

Group 1 Muscles

Body Part	Exercise/Machine, 2 sets	Reps, sets
Chest	Machine chest exercise or free weight chest exercise	15 - 1st 10 - 2nd
Shoulders	Machine shoulder exercise or free-weight shoulder exercise	15 - 1st 10 - 2nd
Triceps	Machine triceps exercise or free weight triceps exercise	15 - 1st 10 - 2nd

Group 2 Muscles

Body Part	Exercise/Machine, 2 sets	Reps, sets
Legs	Machine leg exercise or free-weight leg exercise	15
Calves	Machine or free-weight calf exercise *3 sets for men, 2 sets for women*	15
Back	Machine back exercise or free-weight back exercise	15 - 1st 10 - 2nd
Biceps	Machine biceps exercise or free-weight biceps exercise	15 - 1st 10 - 2nd

STAGE TWO SAMPLE WORKOUT AT HOME

Group 1 Muscles

Body Part	Exercise/Machine, 2 sets each	Reps, sets
Chest	Exercise ball dumbbell press	15 - 1st
	Lying dumbbell fly	10 - 2nd
Shoulders	Bent arm lateral raise,	15 - 1st
	Y shoulder press	10 - 2nd
Triceps	Lying triceps extensions	15 - 1st
	Dumbbell kickbacks	10 - 2nd

Group 2 Muscles

Body Part	Exercise/Machine, 2 sets each	Reps, sets
Legs	Standing reverse lunge	15
	Step-ups	
Calves	3 position calf raises *3 sets for men, 2 sets for women*	15
Back	Exercise ball dumbbell lat row	15 - 1st
	Elbow-out bent-over dumbbell row	10 - 2nd
Biceps	Twisting biceps curl	15 - 1st
	Static 90-degree bicep curl	10 - 2nd

Continue with this regimen for four weeks. After that time, you will have completed a total of six weeks in the gym or at home. You're now ready to learn the concepts that you should follow for the rest of your lifetime of fitness.

STAGE THREE: EXERCISE FOR THE REST OF YOUR LIFE

Stage Three involves working each body part once a week. This is the YOU+ program I recommend for long-term fitness. To exercise each body part once a week, you'll now need to think of your muscles as being in three different groups, instead of two. You'll exercise each group once a week.

PERIODIZATION

Before going into the features of Stage Three, I want to introduce a concept called periodization (also known as periodic training). For our purposes, periodization means changing your workout routine frequently. It also means taking a week off from weight-lifting exercise once every three months.

Periodization first became popular because it was thought to be the reason behind the success of Eastern European athletes during the Cold War. Their training regimen involved altering the emphasis and intensity of the training they did, based on how far out from competition the athletes were. The athletes' progressive training paid off in the 1960 summer Olympics, when the Soviet athletes were very successful, winning 103 medals in total (the United States came in second in the medal count with 71). From that time, the concept of periodization to avoid overtraining and achieve peak performance just in time for important competitions has spread around the world and to every sport.

While you may not be aiming for elite sports performance (I'm certainly not), periodization still applies. It's an excellent way to ensure that you get the most out of the gym without wasting your time, injuring yourself, or overtraining. One aspect of periodization that's extremely important is varying your exercise routine. If you keep doing the same thing the same way over and over again, your body will stop adapting to the demands you put on it. When adaptation stops, you stop getting the full benefits of exercise. Constant variation in your exercise program is necessary.

YOUR STAGE THREE ROUTINE

In strength training, seven parts of the body require regular exercise: chest, back, shoulders, biceps, triceps, calves, and legs. To exercise each body part once a week in Stage Three, divide those seven areas into three different muscle groups. Because you are now exercising fewer muscles at each workout, your sessions will generally be a bit shorter than they were in Stage Two.

To avoid stagnation and reaching training plateaus where you don't make progress, as well as to maximize your insulin efficiency, it's time to add more variety to your program. In addition to varying the individual exercises, it's now time to vary the sequence of muscle groups. So, after a couple of months of doing one set of pairing muscle groups in a particular sequence, switch things around. You may decide to work your legs, calves, and biceps together on one day, your chest and triceps another day, and your back and shoulders on the third day, instead of groupings such as chest/shoulders, biceps/triceps/back, and legs/calves. Whatever combinations you choose, make sure they work each of the seven muscle areas once every week, with adequate rest time between workouts for each area. Mix it up and keep it interesting. Use the YOU+ app and website, which will show you the right way to use new exercises, workout progressions, and combinations, and make sure you're working all of the muscle groups.

In Stage Three, men should do a total of six sets per body part, divided between two or three exercises. The exception to this is that men will perform just three sets for calves, and women should do five sets per body part divided between two exercises. The exception to this is that women will do just two sets of calf exercises. As in Stage Two, exercises for each body part are completed consecutively before moving on to the next body part. Both men and women should use a mix of free weights and exercise machines wherever possible. If you're working out in your home gym, continue to use your free weights and do body weight exercises.

The first set is still 15 repetitions at a weight that is about half of the maximum you could do once. For the upper body, the second set should be a weight you can do 10 times; the third set should also be a weight that you can do only 10 times with excellent effort. If men choose three exercises for two sets each and therefore never reach a third set, the second set of the last two exercises should also be this 10 repetition target. For legs and calves, both the second and third set of any exercise should be 20 repetitions at a weight where the last few are quite a challenge. The rest period between sets is still ideally 90 seconds to two minutes.

To help you plan your strength-training workouts, use the YOU+ app or visit the website. You'll get an individualized program that shows you specifically the exercises, variety, order, and progressions for that week and lets you track your performance. Every exercise is described and illustrated, so you can try new ones and know that you'll be performing them correctly and safely. The YOU+ program is designed to take advantage of the underlying science of exercise and insulin efficiency to give you the best results. Your program is based on your personal needs and abilities—it's flexible and adaptable, and it produces real progress.

A STAGE THREE SAMPLE

An example of the basic approach for Stage Three workouts is below. Over the course of a week, this is a simple way to work all seven different muscle groups in three exercise sessions. Be sure to allow 48 hours rest time between working each particular muscle. At the gym, continue to use machines if you feel comfortable with them, but be sure to move yourself to a combination of free weights and machines—you don't want to get lulled into doing only machines. At home, use your free weights and body weight exercises. The chart below is a starting point—you'll want to vary the exercises regularly to keep your workout fresh.

STAGE THREE BASIC WORKOUT IN THE GYM OR AT HOME

Group 1 Muscles

Body Part	Exercise/Machine	Reps, sets
Chest	Chest machines and free weights	15 - 1st
	free weights and body weight exercises	10 - 2nd
	only if home	10 - 3rd
Shoulders	Shoulder machines and free weights	15 - 1st
	free weights and body weight exercises	10 - 2nd
	only if home	10 - 3rd
	6 sets for men: *choose 2 exercises of 3 sets each or 3 exercises of 2 set each.*	
	5 sets for women: *choose 3 sets of one exercise and 2 sets of another.*	

Group 2 Muscles

Body Part	Exercise/Machine	Reps, sets
Back	Back machines and free weights	15 - 1st
	free weights and body weight exercises	10 - 2nd
	only if home	10 - 3rd
Biceps	Biceps machines and free weights	15 - 1st
	free weights and body weight exercises	10 - 2nd
	only if home	10 - 3rd
Triceps	Triceps machines and free weights	15 - 1st
	free weights and body weight exercises	10 - 2nd
	only if home	10 - 3rd

6 sets for men: *choose 2 exercises of 3 sets each or 3 exercises of 2 set each.*

5 sets for women: *choose 3 sets of one exercise and 2 sets of another.*

Group 3 Muscles

Body Part	Exercise/Machine	Reps, sets
Legs	Leg machines and free weights	15 - 1st
	free weights and body weight exercises	20 - 2nd
	only if home	20 - 3rd

6 sets for men: *choose 2 exercises of 3 sets each or 3 exercises of 2 set each.*

5 sets for women: *choose 3 sets of one exercise and 2 sets of another.*

Body Part	Exercise/Machine	Reps, sets
Calves	Calf machines and free weights	15 - 1st
	free weights and body weight exercises	20 - 2nd
	only if home	20 - 3rd

3 sets for men: *choose 3 sets of one exercise.*

2 sets for women: *choose 2 sets of one exercise.*

EMPHASIZING POWER

For one week of every month during Stage Three, your focus will be on improving your power. You'll do the same exercises, but in a way that increases your muscular power, or the ability to move weight quickly. Power is closely tied to maintaining the ability to do all of the activities you need and want to do in daily life, in any setting.

For your power training week, reduce the weight you use for the second and third set of upper body exercises. The weight should decrease to the point where 15 repetitions of the exercise is a challenge. For your legs and calves, lower the weight to where you can do 25 repetitions. The repetition speed will now be a little faster. As you do your reps, focus on faster movement—pushing or pulling the weight should take one second or less to go from the starting point to the ending point. When I work out, my repetition speed is one to two seconds on all sets anyway, even during periods of heavier lifting. However, the focus on the faster speed and the lighter weights helps to keep the workout fresh and provides the variety that is so necessary for continued improvement. The power week is designated for you on the YOU+ app and website.

VARIETY IS THE SPICE OF THE GYM

Variety keeps your workouts fresh and fun—and it helps you make better progress. Vary the exercises you do for each body part every two or three weeks. You can also vary the rest periods between sets—sometimes 1 minute, sometimes 90 seconds, sometimes 2 minutes—and the number of reps you do. This keeps boredom to a minimum and ensures that your body is adapting all the time. Continuous adaption is essential for keeping your insulin at an efficient level and fighting insulin resistance. As your body continues to adapt, the benefits to your health will range from weight control to disease prevention.

I had a patient named Gerald who had a heart attack. Afterward, he was determined to get into better shape. He went diligently to a cardiac rehab program, where he worked with a trainer and was monitored to make sure his heart was OK as he exercised. Over a period of several months, Gerald's heart stabilized, and he made quite impressive strides. The cardiac rehab program didn't offer a lot of variety, however. He was essentially doing the same workout routine every time he went. Although he continued to go regularly, his progress began to stagnate. After a while, Gerald was so bored and discouraged that he lost the desire to go to the gym.

I recommended a few sessions with a trainer I knew so her could learn how to change things up a bit. After a few sessions with her, Gerald was energized again. He began to get stronger and more energetic, and even improved his blood pressure. He now goes to cardiac rehab for half of his workouts and does the other half on his own to maintain some variety in his resistance exercise regimen. Gerald, like many of my patients, uses the YOU+ app and website to get new ideas for exercises and workouts and to track his progress.

SUPER SLOW—SOMETIMES

Some well-known trainers advocate a "super slow" approach to resistance training. With this method, you take around six to seven seconds to complete one repetition. You'll need to use much less weight to accomplish this; it's harder than you might think. Super slow training does provide a good workout that will certainly exhaust your muscle fibers. It provides some variety from the usual, much faster routine, but I don't recommend making it your main approach. Try it now and then if you want, but the consistent slow speed of the movement doesn't optimize the development of muscle power. Plus, sticking to only one speed lacks the variety you should aim to get from doing various rep speeds and ranges.

AEROBIC EXERCISE

Aerobic (cardio) exercise is valuable for your overall fitness—so valuable that I'll spend all of the next chapter on it. I recommend doing it no more than three or four times a week—not every day. The exception is that it is fine to take a daily walk, which I recommend to many of my patients no matter what other exercise they do. If you wish, combine your aerobic and strength-training workout into one session so that you can get everything done in just three visits to the gym or three home sessions each week. You could do your five-minute warm up, then a few minutes of core exercises, then your sets of weights, finishing with your aerobic exercise. You could do all of these in just about an hour—not a bad use of your time.

If you prefer shorter workouts, you could separate out your cardio days from your weight-training days or do cardio at home (many people prefer this so they can watch TV at the same time). Remember that you need to take a week off from weight training every three months because of periodization—but keep up your regular cardio work even during your off weeks. How to arrange your exercise time is up to you, but find a way. The quality of your life depends on it.

CHAPTER 9
AEROBIC EXERCISE

A LARGE BODY OF medical studies shows that both aerobic and strength exercises are needed for maximum fitness. The most effective way to fight against insulin resistance and maintain a high level of insulin efficiency is to combine your strength training with an aerobic component.

My close friend and training partner is alive today because of aerobic exercise. Mark and I have worked out together for about 15 years. Although he enjoys his weight workouts much more than aerobic exericise, he has been continually faithful to his aerobic work as well. He's an unusually fit guy. And it isn't out of the ordinary for him to do an hour on the stationary bike at its highest resistance level and make it look like a stroll in the park.

One particular weekend, we couldn't work out together because I was out of town with my family, watching my son play in a baseball tournament. In the middle of the night, my cell phone rang. I sprang to answer it so as not to wake my family. It was the emergency room doctor from back home; one of my patients had passed out at the wheel of his car and crashed into a gas station. There were no substantial injuries from the crash, but the heart monitor showed that he was having an abnormal heart rhythm called atrial fibrillation, which was probably responsible for the blackout. It was only after giving me all of this information that he told me the patient's name . . . it was Mark.

I was shocked, to say the least, but the surprises were just beginning. When I arrived at the hospital, the first task was to establish what had caused Mark to pass out at the wheel. We knew from blood tests that he hadn't had a heart attack. When Mark's heart function was evaluated, however, the tests revealed that he had half the heart function he should have had. The next step was a cardiac catheterization, a test that injects dye into the heart arteries; the dye can reveal the presence of blocked arteries. Mark had been a smoker in his early life, but we had no other reason to suspect that lack of blood flow from blocked arteries was a problem. After all, this was a guy who could push the physical limits without difficulty—and someone with blocked heart arteries wouldn't be able to do that, or would at least show some symptoms, such as chest pain, shortness of breath, or unusual fatigue, if he did.

I was in the room when Mark had the catheterization, so I was able to see the pictures as they were shot. My jaw dropped as the first images appeared. Mark's left main artery, the blood vessel that supplies flow to the entire heart, was almost 100 percent blocked. They don't call it the main artery for nothing. A nearly complete blockage to this artery is like shutting off the water at the main pipe, where it comes into your house, as opposed to shutting it off under the sink. In my career, I'd never seen a blockage of this degree in this artery in anyone who was living.

This is where Mark's cardiovascular conditioning comes in. He was in such good condition that his body was able to efficiently use the oxygen from just the trickle of blood that was squeaking through. More amazingly, just a few days before this incident, Mark had done his usual hour on the stationary bike and experienced no symptoms. Without his conditioning, he would be dead, plain and simple.

Thankfully, this story has a happy ending. After bypass surgery, Mark made a complete recovery. His heart function is now back to normal, he feels great, and he's back at the gym training regularly. He has even been able to exceed his fitness benchmarks from before the surgery.

This is one of the major advantages of being fit. When things do go wrong with your health, if you're fit, you're more likely to make a speedy and full recovery. I'm reminded of that basic fact every time I see Mark.

What about you? What would happen to you if your body was slowly developing heart disease or some other life-threatening health problem? Would you be able to overcome it? I'm a great believer in stacking the odds in your favor wherever you can. Fitness means stacking the odds in your favor in terms of preventing disease and also for getting you through it if something does happen to you.

WHY NOT EXERCISE?

Good research has shown that aerobic fitness reduces insulin resistance and improves insulin efficiency. Exercise also reduces the risk of heart disease, certain cancers, stroke, high blood pressure, diabetes, dementia, and bone problems. You would think that this would be enough to get people moving, and yet they don't. Less than 25 percent of Americans get the exercise they need. Why?

In talking to many patients over the years, I've come to believe that there are two main reasons so many people are impervious to advice about exercising. The first is the basic belief that these serious health matters aren't going to happen to them anytime soon. They figure they still have time to start taking their health seriously later. The second belief is that they have come to accept how they currently feel as normal—fatigue, stress, lack of energy, and poor sleep are just the way things are for the average person. People have become so used to feeling flat and lethargic that they don't even realize that this isn't how they are supposed to feel. They simply assume that what they are feeling is normal, or that it's just part of the process of getting older. The average person may indeed feel like this, but this may be so only because the average person isn't that fit. Does this describe you? If so, how's it working for you?

Being unfit is like walking around with 20/40 vision. You can get along just fine, but imagine how it would feel to put on a pair of glasses and gain 20/20 vision. It's a revelation! Suddenly, you'll realize what you've been missing out on. When you look back, you can't believe you functioned with 20/40 vision for so long.

The same goes for fitness. Once you achieve it, you will experience the same sense of clarity about how good you can feel. What fitness means to you will be unique to you. Much depends on your age, size, abilities, and state of health. But in terms of knowing how good you can feel, an answer worthy of a mountaintop philosopher applies: you'll know it when you get there. I can assure you that just as you can see more clearly when you correct a little blurriness in your vision, when you get fit, you will feel, know, and appreciate the difference.

AN AEROBIC PRIMER

I'd like to give you a little background on how aerobic exercise works and how it applies to achieving fitness for you. Having some knowledge of what's physically going on in your body will help you make sense of everything you may have heard about what type of exercise is best for you.

The term "aerobic" refers to how energy is produced to fuel your body. To perform, your muscles need to burn fuel, just as your car needs to burn gasoline to run. The fuel in your muscles is something called adenosine triphosphate, commonly referred to as ATP, which is made, though a complex process, from glucose, fat, or protein. Your car has a fuel tank large enough to hold many gallons of gas. Your body, however, has a tiny fuel tank—you can store only about three ounces of ATP. This is enough for only a few seconds of exercise, which would be like your car only having enough gas to get out of the driveway.

To compensate for this, your body constantly recycles ATP after it's been used—that's how you have enough continuous energy to keep moving. The first five or ten seconds of this replenishing process are assisted by a similar substance called creatine phosphate. To extend the car analogy, the use of creatine phosphate is like a hybrid car engine using electric power in addition to gas. However, after the initial boost from creatine phosphate, your body must find another way to renew its source of ATP.

How your body does this depends on how much oxygen is available. If there's plenty of oxygen, ATP is produced using aerobic metabolism. If there's not enough oxygen, the ATP is produced using anaerobic metabolism.

When you exercise at a moderate level of intensity—where you're not short of breath and can still carry on a conversation—you're providing enough oxygen to your muscles to create ATP aerobically. So, by definition, you're doing aerobic exercise. When you exercise at a higher level of intensity—where you *are* significantly short of breath or can't talk while exercising—you're not providing enough oxygen to your muscles, so ATP is created anaerobically. In this case, by definition, you're doing anaerobic exercise.

In the very early stage of exercise, when you first get started, you briefly do anaerobic exercise until oxygen-rich blood arrives in your muscles.

Anaerobic ATP production isn't very efficient. It also creates a breakdown product called lactic acid, which causes your muscles to feel tired. You've probably experienced this at some point when you had to exert yourself suddenly, such as sprinting to catch a train. You probably just made it—any further and you would have had to stop. You used anaerobic energy during the sprint; when the lactic acid built up, you were forced to stop.

Glucose (our energy currency, or blood sugar) is broken down to drive the anaerobic process. In the absence of oxygen, you can make only two molecules of ATP from every one molecule of glucose. This is similar to your car getting two miles per gallon—not very efficient. Aerobic metabolism, on the other hand, creates 36 ATP molecules for each molecule of glucose. Obviously, aerobic metabolism is much more efficient. Who wouldn't want their car to get 36 miles per gallon instead of 2 miles per gallon? The other big advantage of aerobic metabolism is that it can use fat, not just glucose, to make ATP. That's why aerobic exercise can literally be called fat-burning exercise.

Clearly, there are significant advantages to having your body run efficiently. The goal is to increase your fitness to the point where you are efficiently creating ATP through aerobic, not anaerobic metabolism. If you get out of breath while walking down the block, your body is out of condition and can't make much ATP before it becomes inefficient. If you can walk a mile at a 15-minute-per-mile pace and still talk to your walking partner, your body is in better shape. If you can run a mile, better still.

These different levels of conditioning can be described with the technical term "VO$_2$ max." You may have seen this term if you follow sports closely, as many professional teams use this measure to assess their athletes' conditioning. It's a measure of optimal oxygen uptake—or, in other words, a measure of how fit you are. To put it yet another way, VO_2 max is a measure of maximum exercise capacity. A practical example is my friend Mark, who had an outstanding VO_2 max. Otherwise, he wouldn't have survived the blockage in his heart.

You don't have to know what your VO_2 max number is, but there are good reasons to aim for as high a number as you can reasonably achieve. Fitness is a valuable preventative measure, as was demonstrated in Mark's case. Just as important is the way the body responds, depending on what percentage of your maximum exercise capacity you reach during a workout. One of these big differences in your body's response is which fuel (fat, glucose, or protein) the body uses to make the ATP.

TWO OPPOSING FORCES REVISITED

In chapter one, I touched on the four principles that are key to understanding why the YOU+ program works. Those four principles are insulin efficiency, gastrointestinal hormones, nutrient timing, and the opposing forces of breakdown and repair. Exercise is crucial for the breakdown and repair part.

Your body has two systems that are constantly vying against each other—one that promotes breakdown and one that promotes repair. It takes breakdown within the body (also called inflammation) to signal repair, but we need to ensure that the balance is always shifted toward repair. That way, we can protect ourselves to the greatest extent possible from everything ranging from weight gain to cancer.

This is where exercise comes in like a knight in shining armor. Exercise stimulates the necessary inflammation that will give the signal for repair to happen. Exercise comes with a bonus, however—in fact, you get an unusually high return on your investment. That is, when breakdown is caused by exercise (instead of something else, like being very stressed), the body will have an even greater response in favor of repair. That's the key point to remember: the protective effect prevails when triggered by exercise, and the balance shifts toward repair. The natural chemicals your body creates for repair enter the bloodstream and carry this safeguarding effect throughout the body. Your levels of these positive, healing chemicals remain elevated for hours after exercise.

Importantly, the longer and/or more intense your workout is, the greater the response of the protective process is in return. In other words, the more you do and the more you put into your exercise session, the greater the return on your investment of time and effort.

INFLAMMATION: BAD *AND* GOOD

Everyone has a constant supply of background inflammation going on their body. It can come from many sources, including stress, excess weight, poor diet, sitting too much, and social isolation, among others. Particularly if you're sedentary, you have a constant backdrop of inflammation that damages your body—but you don't get an exercise-induced rush of repair chemicals to soothe it.

We've known ever since the 1950s that heart attacks are directly related to a person's activity level—the more active you are, the lower your chances of having a heart attack. In a study published in 1953, researchers in England looked at the health status of over 31,000 men working in the London transit system. They were searching for the link between what the men did and whether they developed heart disease. They discovered that bus drivers, who sat for most of their work shift, had high rates of heart attacks, often before age 65. Bus conductors, however, were active for most of their shift, because they spent a lot of time climbing up and down the stairs of double-decker buses. The study showed that the bus conductors had a far lower incidence of heart attacks—and that if they did have a heart attack, it occurred later in life and was less likely to be fatal. Perhaps this is why Ralph Kramden, the bus driver from *The Honeymooners* sitcom, yelled so much. All that sitting led to a high level of background inflammation, plus it made him grumpy—and stress increases inflammation. Ralph never got the exercise he needed to release the protective chemicals. Neither did Jackie Gleason, the actor who played Ralph—Gleason had bypass surgery for blocked heart arteries when he was 62.

As another example, a study in *Medicine & Science in Sports & Exercise* showed that compared to those who sit the most, those who stand the most had 54 percent fewer heart attacks. This association held true even after taking into account other risk factors, including diet and smoking. Several similar recent studies support this finding. One 2012 study looked at what happens to people who sit for extended periods of time. It showed that having a desk job could double your risk of a heart attack and could also increase your risk of type 2 diabetes and death from any cause. Today, the average adult spends at least half of his or her time being sedentary—sitting or lying down while awake. The people in the study who spent the most time sitting or lying down had alarmingly higher rates of poor health. Specifically, people who were the most sedentary had a 147 percent increase in the risk of cardiovascular events such as a heart attack; they had a 112 percent greater risk of type 2 diabetes and a 49 percent greater risk of death from any cause.

Stress causes inflammation, which is probably why stress also causes illness; the balance between breakdown and repair stays in breakdown mode for too long. Everyone experiences stress—some more than others. Exercising correctly can counter the undesirable inflammatory effects that stress causes. There is zero doubt that aerobic exercise reduces the risk of heart disease, stroke, certain cancers, obesity, dementia, bone disease, hypertension, and diabetes. People who exercise regularly live longer and enjoy a better quality of life.

HEART OF THE MATTER

The most common cause of death in America is heart disease. The heart muscle is amazing, pumping tirelessly throughout your life. Just like any other muscle, however, the heart must get oxygen and nutrients from the bloodstream to function. But unlike the other muscles in the body, if your heart fails to function properly, you are in grave danger. The main artery to the heart is called the left main artery (you may remember it from Mark's story). The left main artery then splits into various smaller branches that send life-giving oxygen to different parts of the heart. Even the largest of these arteries has only about the same diameter as the stem of a large leaf from a tree in your yard. Not a big lifeline, but your existence depends on it.

Blood course through the coronary (heart-nourishing) arteries your entire lifetime—blood that among other things carries the breakdown and repair chemicals we've been talking about. The coronary arteries are exposed to those chemicals day after day, year after year. It's here where inflammation and breakdown chemicals can wreak havoc. They can cause irritation and damage to the delicate layer of cells that line the blood vessels. The damage then signals even more breakdown and destruction. White blood cells, whose job it is to fight infections, obey the signals that say the blood vessel is being invaded and infiltrate the blood vessel wall. Although the white blood cells are sent to help, what actually happens is that they absorb fat and cholesterol that is flowing by in the bloodstream. As a result, these white blood cells become foamy and filled with gunk—medically, we call this plaque—and they start to clog and narrow the artery. Eventually, the plaque pinches off the artery or narrows it so much that a blood clot forms in it and blocks the blood flow. When that happens, you have a heart attack.

Not all plaque adheres to the artery wall and clogs it—more than half the time, plaque forms just under the lining of the blood vessel inside the wall of the artery and doesn't pinch off the blood flow. These deposits are soft and covered with a fibrous cap. This sort of plaque is just as dangerous as the artery-clogging kind. If the cap breaks, the soft plaque inside spills into the artery, a clot forms, and you have a heart attack.

Either way, the initial irritation from the breakdown chemicals turns the damaged artery into a cholesterol magnet. When you lower the irritation through the lifestyle changes in the YOU+ program, you disrupt this process substantially. You make your arteries more like Teflon than magnets. Traditionally, the field of medicine has focused on reducing what is flowing past by prescribing powerful drugs to lower cholesterol. It makes much more sense just to turn off the magnet. Exercise helps to turn off the magnet.

The term "hardening of the arteries," or atherosclerosis, means the buildup, over time, of plaque. The arteries becomes stiff and less able to respond to changes in your heart rate or blood pressure. Just as the breakdown chemicals play a role in starting the hardening process, they continue after the plaque has formed. When plaque is continually exposed to the breakdown chemicals, more inflammation develops. This inflammation can lead to small cracks or even ruptures in the plaque.

This is a disaster, because the body thinks it needs to close the rupture, just as it would if you cut your knee. A clot forms and blocks the flow of blood through the artery. You have a heart attack that cuts off the oxygen supply to the heart muscle downstream; and without oxygen, the muscle begins to die. The severity and survivability of the heart depends on what part of the heart is blocked off and how large an area is affected. The greater the blocked area, the bigger the heart attack is and the more heart muscle that dies. The more heart muscle that dies, the less likely you are to have a good recovery.

As you visualize that scenario, remember the body's response to exercise. By exercising, you create and distribute a substantial amount of soothing and repair resources. Every time you exercise, the protective process flows through all the arteries of your heart and fights back against the sequence that leads to hardening of the arteries and a heart attack.

HOW MUCH AEROBIC EXERCISE DO YOU NEED?

Clearly, there are considerable benefits to aerobic exercise, but how much do you have to do to protect yourself? Many studies have tried to answer this question. It comes down to three main variables:

- The amount of time you exercise
- The intensity of your exercise
- How often you exercise

If the idea of intense, sweaty exercise fills you with dread, you'll be glad to hear that you don't even need to break a major sweat to achieve some benefits. The studies that support this finding suggest that even exercising at the intensity of a moderately paced walk is helpful. Given the amount of study on the subject, I am convinced that an exercise as simple as walking for as little as 20 minutes three times per week can be beneficial. There is even data that indicates you don't need to do 20 minutes at one time. Ten-minute increments, so long as they add up to the total time, are helpful and may be as good as or better than doing it all at once. Leisure-time activities like golf (if you walk the course) or gardening—if you do these activities often enough—also have benefit. Even cleaning the house is a form of exercise.

Overwhelming evidence, however, says that the more exercise you do, the significantly greater the benefit. I hope this is what you strive for. The more effort the exercise requires, the greater the return on the investment in regard to the soothing repair substances that are released. The more soothing substances you have floating around your body, the greater the amount of allies you have to protect you from things like heart disease.

Don't get me wrong: I would much rather have you do light exercise like walking, golfing, or gardening than none at all. But if you're already doing this, or if you've progressed from being sedentary to achieve regular light exercise, think about doing more. You've probably already noticed some benefits from your exercise. Isn't it time to strive for even greater benefits?

If you're going to take the time to do aerobic exercise, make it count! Clearly, you'll want to find your personal balance between doing so little that it's barely worth your time, and doing so much that you hate it. When exercise becomes so much of an effort that you dread doing it, you won't stick to it. Additionally, if it's something that results in injury, you're going to stop doing it—and you may never go back.

When you start exercising beyond just light activity, you have a lot to gain. One advantage is that it will increase your aerobic capacity as measured by that technical term VO_2 max.

Remember that this capacity was significant in Mark's survival because it has to do with the delivery and use of oxygen by the body. You want your oxygen capacity to be as high as possible. When you put more effort into your exercise program by increasing your aerobic activity, your oxygen capacity can improve by up to 30 percent.

Many studies correlate levels of fitness and the risk of death from all causes. One measure of fitness often used is something called a MET (metabolic equivalent of task, or just metabolic equivalent), which is a measurement that reflects your baseline use of oxygen. We use METs as way to express the intensity and energy expenditure of an activity, or, to put it more simply, METs measure how hard your body is working. Just sitting quietly takes one MET. Walking at a moderate speed takes about 3.5 METs. How many multiples of that baseline number of 1 MET that you can achieve—by walking on a treadmill, for instance— is a good indicator of your fitness level.

In a landmark study published in the *New England Journal of Medicine* in 2002, researchers looked at how fitness levels related to death rates. The baseline fitness level for participants was found to be 7 METs for older men and 10 METs for younger men.

The results of this important study were both astounding and eye-opening. Within each group, when compared to each other, each extra MET a subject could achieve lowered his risk of dying from any cause by about 12 percent over the next six years. I want to emphasize *any cause*. That includes stroke, heart disease, cancer, or anything else you can name.

Again, no matter where you start, each extra MET you can achieve over your baseline by improved conditioning *reduces your risk of death from any cause* by 12 percent. If you start at 4 and go to 9, you have reduced your risk of dying from any cause by 60 percent. If you start at 9 and go to 11, you have lowered your odds by another 24 percent. This isn't true just for men. A study of over ten thousand women showed similar results.

Another large investigation, published in the *Journal of the American Medical Association* in 1989, also had impressive results. The study was conducted by the Institute for Aerobics Research and the Cooper Clinic, and had over thirteen thousand healthy participants. The researchers looked at their physical fitness and overall death rates over an eight-year period. When the least fit men were compared to the fittest men, the least fit were more than three times as likely to die over the eight years. Among women, the least fit were over four and a half times more likely to die when compared to the most fit during the time they were followed. This study also showed that becoming even a little more fit was helpful, but the higher your aerobic capacity, the greater the overall benefit.

In essence, if you achieve these higher fitness levels, you are only about one-third to one-half as likely to die prematurely compared to people who never reach these higher levels of fitness. Your life will be of better quality, with more energy, less chronic illness, and more ability to perform the activities of daily living easily. This sounds like a pretty fair trade for your exercise time. These studies also illustrate that the advantages gained from exercise, including its protective power, can't be accomplished with just light activities like leisurely walking, gardening, or playing golf. To give you an idea of what can be achieved, I have a 50-year-old female patient who came to me with atypical chest pain. Her cardiac stress test was normal, but her exercise capacity was poor, which made her decide it was definitely time to get in shape. She began following the YOU+ principles. A year later, when we repeated the stress test, she achieved an amazing 17 METs—and the results were completely normal. (It also turned out that her chest pain had been caused by acid reflux.) That compares extremely well to the average of 7 to 10 METs cited above. My patient was 50 years old and had never really exercised when she began the program, showing that a high level of fitness can be achieved through the YOU+ program, regardless of your age or level of fitness when you start.

CHAPTER 10
THE YOU+ AEROBIC EXERCISE PLAN

AEROBIC EXERCISE, ALSO KNOWN as cardio exercise, doesn't require the same level of planning and precision as resistance exercise to reap the full benefits. That doesn't mean it's less important for your fitness.

Aerobic exercise by definition means exercise that increases your heart rate. As with any exercise program, if you have any doubt about your safety when you exercise, check with your doctor before beginning.

WHAT AEROBIC EXERCISE SHOULD YOU DO?

What type of aerobic exercise you do is really only limited by your imagination and your personal preferences. Aerobic work can include pretty much any physical activity, so long as you're moving your large muscle groups continuously.

The old aerobics standbys include activities such as walking or running on a treadmill or outdoors, using exercise machines like an elliptical or stair stepper, and riding a stationary bike or a real one outside. But aerobic exercise can also be dance, swimming, trampoline, or cross-country skiing. If you're more athletically inclined, what about rollerblading or ice skating? Many gyms offer spinning, a form of stationary bike exercise set to music. Your gym probably also offers all sorts of other aerobic exercise classes featuring a wide variety of music or movement styles—you should easily find one that you like or that fits your schedule. Maybe kickboxing or Zumba is more your style. The point is, you can always find some form of aerobic exercise that you can do and enjoy. I encourage you to change your aerobic routine regularly to keep it from getting stale. Don't be afraid to try something new!

Whatever you choose, I recommend that you include a low-impact activity as part of your regular exercise. Low-impact means that you don't land on your feet with your full body weight on a hard surface—this can increase your risk of injury. Running and many aerobics classes are higher impact and shouldn't make up your entire aerobic activity. Besides, it's always better to vary your aerobic workout so you don't get bored by doing the same thing all the time. Playing music or listening to the radio or podcasts through headphones or watching the gym TVs are also helpful to keep your interest. If you have an exercise machine in your home, use your headphones, or position it in front of the TV. If you use it during a show you were planning to watch anyway, you leverage your time for additional benefit. The bottom line is that if you want to be healthy and energetic, you just have to do aerobic activity consistently.

After a while, your aerobic exercise will become a habit, part of your routine, just like other parts of your schedule. In your daily life, you make time for other people; make sure you pencil in time for yourself as well. Make an appointment with yourself and keep it. Exercising with a friend makes it much more enjoyable—the time passes quickly, and you may actually find yourself having fun. Plus, if someone else is counting on you to be there, you're much more likely to show up.

AEROBIC EXERCISE: HOW OFTEN, HOW LONG, HOW INTENSE?

I recommend that you do aerobic exercise at least three times each week. If you do it less than twice a week, you won't develop much additional aerobic fitness. The real threshold for improvement is three times a week. If you exercise four or five days weekly, you'll get some additional but smaller incremental improvement. More than five times weekly has a tiny effect on increasing your level of fitness, but your risk of an injury goes up. To prevent overtraining, try to keep your total days of exercise (including resistance training) to, at most, four or five days per week. This is not to say you couldn't or shouldn't engage in light activities like walking on your off days.

How long your cardio workouts need to be depends on the intensity of the workout. For general fitness, lower-intensity exercise for longer periods is essentially equal to higher-intensity exercise for shorter periods. Research suggests that the total energy expended—not how slowly or quickly you expend it—is the key factor. In other words, if lower intensity/longer time is equal to higher intensity/shorter time in terms of energy expended, you get equal benefit.

I recommend doing cardio for 20 to 30 minutes for the average person. This time includes a few minutes for warming up and a few minutes for cooling down. If you want to go longer, that's fine, but 30 minutes maximum is enough for achieving higher fitness.

Higher intensity in a shorter time frame may be more convenient time-wise, but most people do better in the long haul with longer duration at a more sustainable level of effort. The duration doesn't necessarily have to be done all at once for you to benefit—the concept of total energy expended comes into play. If you use the same amount of energy in three 10-minute sessions that you would in one 30-minute session, you will accomplish very much the same thing. Several shorter sessions might be a useful approach to start with, but I know from experience with my patients that you will build your exercise capacity faster if you go with one longer session.

YOUR LEVEL OF EFFORT

The outcome of exercise depends largely on the intensity of the workout. The most widely used measure of intensity is your heart rate. This involves continually checking your pulse to see if you are in your "target range" as you do your workout.

Constantly checking your pulse rate is distracting and takes away some of the fun of your workout. And there's more to your aerobic exercise than aiming for a particular number. It's much easier and more practical to rate yourself on how you perceive your own level of effort, using a well-established and studied scale. Rating your effort is particularly useful because it takes different levels of conditioning and ability into account. For example, two people may be exercising on stationary bikes at the same level of resistance. One may assess his level of perceived effort as moderate while the other, who is less conditioned, may assess his level of perceived effort as high, even though they are doing the same thing.

As the second person improves his fitness, his current level of exercise will require less effort. Now, to achieve the same perceived level of effort, he will have to increase the resistance on the bike, or he'll have to cycle for longer. By maintaining the same level of effort as your fitness improves, your exercise routine is self-regulating. This is the best way to achieve long-term results.

The standard exertion scale used by doctors, physical therapists, and others is called the Borg Rating of Perceived Exertion (RPE). For some reason, the scale starts at 6 and goes to

20. Although it's widely used, the Borg scale just feels odd—6 on the scale means sitting doing nothing, while 20 is maximal effort. My patients find it more logical to use a scale that runs from 1 to 15 instead. The rankings for each step on the Willey exertion scale are in the chart below.

WILLEY EXERTION SCALE

1–2	very, very light
3–4	very light
5–6	fairly light
7–8	moderate
9–10	hard
11–12	very hard
13–14	very, very hard
15	maximum effort

The level of effort (intensity) you should aim for is between 7 and 10 on this scale. Remember, if you choose to work out at the lower ranges, you will need to exercise for longer to achieve the same expenditure of energy. Your workout will take longer, closer to the 30-minute end of the range. If you exercise at an intensity closer to the 10 benchmark, you don't need to go as long to get the same improvement in aerobic capacity. You don't have to choose the same intensity level every time. You'll simply feel better on some days than on others. Adjust your effort accordingly.

Working with the Willey scale has another advantage. People who exercise at a perceived effort level of about 8 tend to stick with exercise better than those who go too low or too high. If you already use a heart rate monitor to track your level of intensity, studies have shown that the 7 to 10 range of effort correlates well with the target heart rates ranges recommended by most experts.

The standard heart rate target formula is based on your age. This formula is: (220 minus your age) x 55 to 90 percent. To illustrate how calculations based on heart rate work in practice, let's look at an example. If you're 60 years old, subtract your age from 220 to get 160. Next, multiply 160 by 55 percent (0.55) to get 88 for your lower range. Then take 160 (220 minus 60) and multiply it by 90 percent (0.90) to get 144 for the higher end of your range. Obviously, the ranges will change as you age.

The perceived effort technique, however, doesn't change since it's determined by your personal fitness level, not your age plugged into a formula. It's much easier to measure where you fall on the scale of perceived effort than to spend your work-out checking your heart rate. If you're exercising at a perceived effort level of between 7 and 10, you're where you need to be.

When you first start doing regular aerobic exercise, I suggest you check your heart rate once in a while just to be sure that the perceived level you think you're working at does genuinely fall into your desired heart rate range. If it doesn't, rethink how you're rating your perceived effort level so that being in the 7 to 10 range does match up with your heart rate. Once you see that your perceived effort level and heart rate correlate accurately, you can leave the constant pulse-checking to others. If you don't have a heart rate monitor to do this occasional check in the beginning, you don't need to rush out and buy one. Most aerobic machines in your local gym have built-in heart rate monitors. All you have to do is hold the sensors on the handles for a few moments as your exercise and you'll see your heart rate on the display.

HOW TO PROGRESS

If you're new to aerobic exercise, I recommend that you start with walking at a reasonable pace. The YOU+ plan is for a lifetime of fitness—you don't need to rush in and do something that makes you sore the first day or that turns out to be something you don't enjoy. After you've been walking regularly for a couple of weeks, branch out into other activities, using the Willey exertion scale as your guide. If you've been a regular exerciser, you can skip walking and proceed right into the exertion scale. Either way, remember, it's not about how much you can do or how long you can go; it's about how much effort you expend doing it.

Using the Willey exertion scale also makes it easy to progress at the correct pace for you. All you have to do is keep up the same level of effort. As your body builds better aerobic capacity, you will naturally be doing more at the same level of perceived exertion, and you will progress appropriately. Just listen to your body; it will lead you well.

WHAT ABOUT WEIGHT LOSS?

So far in this book, we've covered the five parts of an exercise prescription: what exercise to do, how frequently, how long, how intense, and how to progress. The focus has been on increasing your aerobic capacity and improving how well and how long you live. The reality, however, is that for many people, the driving reason for doing aerobic exercise is to achieve their desired weight. While aerobic exercise can help with weight loss, that's not the main reason for doing it. *Exercise improves how well and how long you live, even if you don't lose weight.*

One of my patients wanted to lose weight. She started doing regular aerobic workouts, spending up to two hours in the gym every session but not really changing her diet much or doing resistance exercise. After three months, she was pretty disheartened because her weight hadn't budged. She was so fit, however, that she was able to climb Mt. Kilimanjaro and raise a lot of money for a charity. That's the important point about exercise. It's beneficial even if your weight doesn't change. If your focus, however, is on weight loss, then there are superior ways to achieve that outcome.

THE BEST WAY TO BURN FAT

The most common question my patients ask me is, "What's the best aerobic exercise, at what intensity, for fat burning?" The answer is that what fuel you burn for energy (fat, protein, or glucose) isn't the prime factor in successful weight loss.

The main fuels the body uses during aerobic exercise are fat and glucose. Remember, glucose is the form of sugar that is the body's energy currency. When you exercise at a light intensity, your body burns a higher percentage of fat than glucose as its fuel. At light intensity (around 6 or less on the exertion scale), your body has plenty of oxygen available, so the exercise is aerobic. Your energy demand leaves enough time for ATP to be made from fat. As your exercise becomes more moderate, around 8 on the scale, your body will burn roughly equal amounts of glucose and fat and still be highly aerobic. The body can do this because it takes more time and oxygen to convert fat to ATP than it does to convert glucose to ATP. When you are exercising at a higher intensity—10 or so on the exertion scale—you need more oxygen, so there's less to spare for the fat conversion process. Your body still burns some fat at this level, but it mostly turns to glucose instead. As you continue to increase the intensities of exercise, your body burns glucose as its exclusive source of fuel.

At this point, you might be thinking that you should always exercise at the lower intensity levels to achieve the greatest fat loss. The problem is, at low intensity, even though a high percentage of calories burned are from fat, you just don't burn as many calories overall. The calories burned when you exercise at moderate intensity have a lower percentage from fat, but you will burn more calories overall than with light exercise. You will also end up burning more total fat calories this way, so focus on moderate exertion for maximum weight-loss results.

Let's look at an example. Say you exercise at light intensity and burn 120 calories. About 90 of those calories will come from fat. If you exercise at moderate intensity and burn 180 calories, half of those calories will still come from fat. So, you've burned 90 fat calories but have also burned 60 calories more in total. The more calories you burn during exercise, the more the body can later dip into fat stores to make up the deficit you created— and the greater the deficit, the greater the dip. In addition, you'll increase your metabolism (calories burned) to a greater degree and for a longer time after your exercise session if you work at a more vigorous intensity. As you get into better shape, you are doing more at the same level of perceived exertion on the scale. What you now perceive as moderate intensity is actually more vigorous than the moderate intensity you used to perceive. You're now burning more total calories (and fat calories) than you did before.

INTERVAL TRAINING FOR FAT BURNING

Interval training—varying the intensity of your exercise within an aerobic session—is another approach to fat burning. It's supported by solid research, and indications are that interval training may turn out to be the best approach to aerobic fitness. Varying your intensity within a session of aerobic exercise can apparently accomplish even more than exercising at a constant intensity. Interval training has been shown to increase calorie burning over standard aerobic training during the exercise session *and* for a period of time long after the exercise is over.

One effective pattern for varying your intensity is switching between exercise intensities that are 6 or 7 on the Willey exertion scale with intensities that go up to 10 or 11 on the scale. Switch every two to five minutes between the two intensities. In fact, you don't even have to switch intensities with the same exercise. You could go hard on the stationary bike for five minutes, for example, and then switch to the treadmill for an easy five minutes. You could swim for a few minutes, then walk in the water for a few minutes. Even if you're walking, you could walk as fast as you can for five minutes, then go back to your usual pace. Make it up as you go along! Don't limit yourself to set intensities, duration of intensity, or specific rest periods between each interval. The bottom line is that interval training is a good addition to your repertoire. Not only is it good for calorie burning, but it also gives you another way to mix things up and keep it interesting.

TIMING AEROBIC EXERCISE FOR WEIGHT LOSS

My patients often ask me what time of day is best for maximum weight loss from aerobic exercise. My answer is that I'd rather have you do it any time than not do it at all. If you want to try to squeeze out a time advantage, it's possible that early evening or after you do your strength training may maximize weight loss.

Although working out first thing in the morning is frequently recommended, I believe that it's overrated. The theory is that your glucose stores are lower in the morning, so you may draw on fat as a higher percentage of your workout fuel. It's the total amount of calories burned based on intensity that's the most important factor, however. If you work out to a high intensity in the morning, you're still going to burn glucose, not fat.

There's also the possibility that your body will eat into muscle stores if you do cardio first thing, because your body will utilize protein for energy. The biggest advantage of morning cardio, in reality, is that you get it done and set the tone for your day. If you've already worked out in the morning, you may be less likely to eat unhealthy foods later in the day and ruin all your good work.

Some recent data suggests that early evening workouts have the advantage. It's possible that doing your cardio at this time will increase your calorie burning for longer after you exercise. The improved effect of evening training isn't likely, however, to be equal to the extended calorie burning capabilities of interval training. Also, some people find that an early evening workout is so energizing that they have trouble sleeping, although my patients tell me that after a week or two, they get used to the evening schedule and the sleep issues vanish.

The other frequently cited optimal exercise time is after strength training. Your glucose stores are reduced after strength training because you worked your muscles first. However, I think there are even bigger advantages to be gained by doing cardio after strength training than just the type of fuel you use. Since the energy for strength workouts comes almost entirely from stored glucose, if you do strength training first, the energy stores are still available for the strength workout. In other words, you haven't depleted your stores from doing your cardio first. You will then be better able to safely focus greater effort into your strength training and then maximize the fat-burning effects of the cardio that you do afterward.

Doing cardio after strength training also benefits hormone responses. Naturally enhancing hormone levels is a part of achieving optimal fitness. Although these levels are particularly integrated with strength training and nutrition and are positively affected by the methodologies you have read about, aerobic train-ing is also an important element. For example, studies suggest that your level of growth hormone may be enhanced if you do your cardio after, rather than before, strength training. Growth hormone is very important for maintaining strength and lean-ness, so this approach may be valuable.

If there's one single answer to when and how to do your cardio, it may well be to do interval cardio after strength training in the evening. You'll burn the greatest number of fat and total calories, and you may get a hormonal advantage as well.

CHAPTER 11
CORE STABILITY AND STRENGTH

CORE TRAINING HAS BECOME widely accepted as an important part of fitness, and with good reason. Core stability and strength are vital to how your body moves. Everything you do, every movement you make, originates and flows from strong core muscles. Your core supports your spine and helps keep your body balanced and stable. It provides a center of gravity and allows for better performance of movement. A healthy core provides better coordination, breathing, digestion, posture, and protection from injury, and fights against back pain.

So what exactly is the core? The core comprises the muscles around your trunk and pelvis. These muscles include the rectus abdominis (the six-pack muscle) that people tend to focus on, but the core is much more than that. The other critical muscles have names such as the transversus abdominis, obliques, erector spinae, gluteus medius, and gluteus maximus. You can see from the length of this list that a lot more is involved in core training than just your six pack. The muscles involved run the length of your torso.

By now you may be getting concerned that your core stability and strength routine is going to demand even more of your workout time. The good news is that just a few minutes of your workout will effectively train your core and let you reap the benefits.

In this chapter, we'll also briefly cover the topics of balance and stretching. Although balance and stretching aren't limited to core muscles, this is an appropriate place to discuss these important additions to your workout, as they will help deliver even better results. Core stability, strength, balance, and stretching yield a disproportionate benefit from the small additional time required to address these areas.

I remember when I first really understood that core muscles were separate from general conditioning and that they required specific attention. I was a medical resident and, despite the long hours, was quite regular in my workout routine. I particularly enjoyed weight training, but I did cardiovascular training as well. My cardio exercises were mainly a carry-over from my high school days of cross country and track. I thought that I had it all pretty well covered, although not everyone who knew me agreed.

My wife is a physical therapist, and she had a background in dance before attending PT school. Through her training, she was well versed in matters of core stability and was fond of telling me how I ought to pay more attention to my core training. I probably didn't give it the credence I should have, for two reasons. First, I already thought I was in reasonably good shape. And second, at my young age, I still thought that what I was taught in school was the aggregate of all the subjects I needed to know. They didn't mention anything about the core in medical school. At the same time, however, I was maturing as a physician and was beginning to realize that there were many other things that were important; I just didn't know enough about them yet.

At any rate, one day my wife challenged me to perform some simple core exercises and hold the positions for what seemed to be a reasonable and doable period of time. Needless to say, I didn't do nearly as well as I thought I would. I had learned what physical therapists, dancers, and many others had known for a long time. The core needs special attention to yield its considerable benefits.

CORE STABILITY AND STRENGTH

A good place to start is where I did, by testing your existing core stability and strength. Start by taking a few minutes to see how you do on a basic core task. This particular task is one that most everyone can do for a little while. Doing it will give you a baseline and also give you a way to measure your improvement over time. All you need is a flat surface (the floor) and an easy-to-read timing device, such as a watch with a second hand or the stopwatch on your phone.

Place the watch or timer where it's easy to see, and then get into the basic plank position, which is really no more than a modified push-up position. The difference between the plank and a push-up position is that you support yourself on your forearms and toes instead of your hands and toes. Place your forearms flat on the floor, from your fingertips to your elbows, directly beneath your shoulders for support. Hold your body straight; don't arch or round your back. Your body should form a straight line from your head to your feet—imagine it as a plank of wood.

Once you're in position with your back straight, hold the plank for as long as you can, up to 60 seconds. If you're able to hold for 60 seconds in the initial plank position, try to raise your right foot off the ground a few inches. If you can hold that for 10 seconds, then put your right foot back down and try to lift your left foot off the ground for 10 seconds and then place it back down. If at any point you can't complete the task, even if it's shortly after starting the initial plank position, stop and record how far you made it for future comparison.

If you're still going, try to raise your right arm off the ground a few inches and hold for 10 seconds. If you have success there, then put your right arm back down and try to hold your left arm off the ground for 10 seconds. The final step for the occasional person who makes it this far would be to put your left arm back on the ground and hold the basic plank position for another 30 seconds. Your goal is not necessarily to reach a certain point, but rather to continue to improve over time. Ideally, you'll eventually be able to complete the entire task. The times or positions can be adjusted, but this is a good general starting guideline for assessing the strength of your core.

Another way to evaluate yourself before getting started is to look at your posture. Good core health, along with strength training, will improve your posture and help protect you from injuries and many sources of pain, especially back and neck pain. Basically, good posture is having the body in proper alignment as it relates to gravity. You should be able to form an imaginary line through your ankles, knees, hips, shoulders, and ears.

A simple way to check your posture is the wall test. As the name implies, all you need is a wall. Stand with your back against the wall; the back of your head should also touch the wall. Place your heels six inches from the wall. Put one hand between your lower back and the wall, and then between your neck and the wall. If the spaces between your body and the wall are only about two inches, your posture is quite good. If the spaces are greater, core exercises will help improve your posture.

The advantages of these self-evaluations are that they can be done anywhere, which is very helpful for core exercises. The plank test is itself a good core exercise, as are numerous others that are also easy to do at home and provide the different movements necessary to get the whole core involved in your workout. Machines and gym equipment add even more choices to work your core.

The majority of core exercises are really abdominal exercises, but it's important to also work the non-abdominal core muscles, including some back and hip muscles and the gluteus muscles. I recommend doing four core exercises per workout. There are many, many variations of core exercises. Choose one for your lower abs, one for your upper abs, one for your oblique (side) abs, and one general core stability exercise, such as the plank. As with the rest of your workout, vary the core exercises you do and the order in which you do them. Mix things up every couple of weeks, or more often if you prefer. I recommend little, if any, rest between sets of core exercises. I typically move right from one into the next.

The YOU+ app and website have lots of great information and videos showing core exercises, and you can also follow an individualized core exercise training plan that will help you get the most out of your core exercise in the most efficient manner.

PILATES

A popular method of promoting core strength is Pilates. Although the growth in Pilates studios is a recent phenomenon, the exercise system has been around for over a century. It was developed by Joseph Pilates, a German-born physical trainer who went to England in 1912 to teach self-defense to Scotland Yard detectives. When World War I broke out, he was interned as an enemy alien in Britain. He made the most of his time by developing a form of exercise that used minimal equipment and focused on the core muscles of the torso. After the war, Pilates returned to Germany and taught his methods to dancers there. In 1926, Pilates immigrated to the United States, eventually opening a fitness studio in New York City. Not coincidentally, he was located near the New York City Ballet; his methods soon became very popular with dancers. Pilates' method remained fairly confined to this clientele until after his death in 1967. In the 1970s, a Pilates studio in Beverly Hills gained popularity with Hollywood celebrities, and the method began to gain momentum. Today, Pilates is a mainstream approach to core exercise practiced by some 10 million Americans.

Pilates is an exercise routine that works the core while also building strength, flexibility, endurance, and coordination—without adding muscle mass. Pilates requires the involvement of your mind as well as your body to focus on your breathing rhythm in combination with your body movements. Pilates movements emphasize spinal and pelvic alignment as well as posture. Most exercises are done on a mat, but machines are available in many studios.

A Pilates workout is a sequence of exercises with smooth, continuous movements that flow, one into the next, in a natural progression. One of the advantages of Pilates is that almost anyone can do it regardless of their initial conditioning level. Beginners start with basic exercises and can progress to additional exercises and more difficult positions, just as with the plank. The goal is to employ smooth movements; Joseph Pilates designed his exercises to flow like a dance.

If you would like to try Pilates, find a well-qualified instructor who has completed several hundred hours of training. Some gyms and exercise studios send their personal trainers on a weekend course to become certified, but clearly this isn't ideal training. Many of my patients have tried Pilates and have enjoyed it. If you think Pilates could help you stick with a program to improve your core, give it a try.

FLEXIBILITY AND STRETCHING

Just as core strength is fundamental to fitness, so is flexibility. One of the first things we all do when we wake up is stretch out in some way, perhaps by extending the arms as we yawn. Animals do it, too. You've seen how a dog or cat gets up from a nap and stretches. Stretching inherently feels good—we instinctively know it's good for us.

Stretching is closely related to fitness, but maybe not in the way you think. In the medical literature, our ideas about stretching have evolved significantly, but some deeply ingrained—and false—ideas about stretching are still followed. You've almost certainly been told about the importance of stretching before you work out. The conventional wisdom is that pre-workout stretching can prevent injury. Whether this is actually true is an area of contention and controversy. The research is trending toward the idea that the old stretching standard does *not* prevent injury.

In the past, and even today, the type of stretching recommended for injury prevention is known as passive or static stretching. A good example of passive stretching is propping your leg up on a bench. While some studies suggest that passive stretching may help prevent injury, many more indicate it does nothing whatsoever to prevent injuries.

Studies of how stretching affects performance have also cast doubt on conventional thinking. A review in the *Clinical Journal of Sports Medicine* looked at the effects on performance from doing the recommended passive stretching before the activity. The authors reviewed 23 high-quality journal articles and found that 22 of them showed no benefit on multiple performance parameters. In contrast, they looked at nine studies of regular stretching—stretching done regularly for its own sake, not as a way to prepare for an activity. Seven studies showed a benefit from regular stretching, not just stretching before an activity.

The other two studies were unclear—they only looked at one isolated aspect of running performance. This review suggests that passive (static) stretching before an activity is pretty useless, but regular stretching as part of a fitness routine can be helpful because it maintains the full range of motion.

The inefficiency of static stretching as it relates to performance makes sense when you consider how muscles and tendons work together. It all has to do with how energy is distributed by these structures. Tendons are tough, fibrous tissues that attach muscles to bones. Think of your tendon as a nail and your muscle as a piece of wood. A hammer hitting the nail and driving it into the wood is a transfer of energy. The stretched tendon is like a softer nail, made of hard rubber instead of steel. The more energy that gets to the muscle, the better your performance will be. When you stretch by the standard static method, the tendon is more of a shock absorber. It will absorb more energy, leaving less for the muscle and less for your performance. The unstretched tendon absorbs less energy, which means more energy is transferred to the muscle for the work at hand, and hence provides optimal performance.

DYNAMIC FLEXIBILITY

Flexibility has several components. Passive flexibility is the ability to assume a position and hold it by a means other than your own muscular power. An example of passive flexibility would be the ability to prop your leg up on a bench—the bench, not your muscles, holds up your leg. Active flexibility is holding a stretched position using your own muscle power. An example would be holding your leg up to stretch it without the bench to prop it up. The third type of flexibility is dynamic flexibility—that's the type of flexibility I want to emphasize.

Dynamic flexibility is the ability to use your muscles to move a joint through its full range of motion—the entire spectrum of movement the joint was designed to have. Of course, this varies from joint to joint. For example, your knee joint can move in only two directions. You should be able to extend your knee all the way out to a straight-leg position, as well as bend it backward so your heel touches your backside. This is the knee's full range of motion.

Dynamic flexibility is most closely related to what you actually do when you move your body from day to day. Achieving a good range of motion is one of the key benefits to having good dynamic flexibility. Having a full range of motion from good flexibility will help prevent imbalances, which are a frequent cause of debility and/or pain. For example, decreased range of motion in the hamstring muscles in the back of your thighs (sometimes called "tight" hamstrings) is a common contributor to back pain.

Being able to move your body to its fullest ability is very helpful for your fitness and the activities of daily living. Would you buy a TV that came equipped to get hundreds of channels but got only 75? You should apply the same standard to your body. Dynamic stretching will help you achieve this.

DYNAMIC STRETCHING

Dynamic stretching is using your own muscle power to move a body part in a controlled manner through its full range of motion. Some examples of dynamic stretching would be swinging your arms in large circles, jogging slowly while focusing on kicking your knees higher and higher, or backpedaling with progressively longer steps. Dynamic stretching can also be activity specific, such as doing a weight-lifting exercise with an extremely light weight for a number of repetitions before actually performing the exercise with the weight you would typically use. A large number of studies support the use of dynamic stretching in competitive sports because it optimizes performance. For our purposes, dynamic stretching increases your range of motion, helps you warm up, and increases blood flow to help you feel your best during exercise.

WHAT TO DO BEFORE EXERCISE

No matter what sort of exercise you're planning to do, I believe that warming up with five minutes of aerobic activity is necessary to elevate your body temperature and increase blood flow to your muscles. Follow the aerobic exercise with some dynamic stretching that's specific to whatever activity you are about to do. For example, before playing tennis, you might swing your racquet lightly for a minute or so through the full range of motion you are going to use. This is efficient and takes very little time. If you're going to do cardio exercise, such as run on a treadmill, do some dynamic stretching for the first five minutes by going at a much easier pace of whatever intensity level you're planning.

Before you begin your resistance or strength-training exercises, do a five-minute aerobic warm-up followed by dynamic stretching. Using an extremely light weight, go through the full range of motion for the first exercise for that body part you are about to perform. Fifteen repetitions is a good and simple way to accomplish this. In Chapter 8, you learned that the first set of any exercise should be 15 reps at a weight that is about 50 percent of what you think you could lift once. This first ultra-light dynamic stretching weight should be done before that first set. It's a nice transition to the heavier resistance exercise.

WHAT TO DO AFTER EXERCISE

The best time to engage in the more traditional (passive or static) stretching is after you've finished your exercise routine. After a workout, passive stretching as part of the cooling-down process may help reduce post-workout soreness or stiffness. It also helps the muscle "remember" its pre-workout length so it can optimize development and performance. Remember, seven out of nine studies showed a performance benefit of regular stretching as opposed to standard stretching right before an activity. Outside of performance, I think stretching just makes you feel better, both physically and mentally.

Some trainers advocate daily stretching as part of a fitness regimen, but I have found that stretching only after your three weekly exercise sessions works well for most people. If you like to stretch every day, be careful of overstretching, which increases your risk of injury. You should not be sore the next day from stretching alone. If you are, this is a sign that you need to back off.

I recommend doing two stretching sets for each of the body parts you just used in your workout. You may also find this to be a good time to do whole-body stretching to get the maximum out of your body's abilities. If you do whole-body stretching, start with the back, then do the neck and upper body, and end with the lower body.

How long to hold the stretch isn't clear from the medical literature. From looking at the data, a stretch of 10 to 30 seconds seems reasonable. A couple of reasons are probably behind that time frame. The first is the stretch reflex. This is the body's response to a muscle being stretched. It reflexively contracts the stretched muscle to resist the force upon it. The more quickly you stretch, the more vigorous the resistive response is. This is why you should always stretch slowly. After a time, the muscle gets used to the new length and the stretch reflex lessens.

The other reaction is called the lengthening reaction, which is essentially the opposite of the stretch reflex. When the muscle is stretched, the lengthening reaction keeps it from contracting and helps it to relax—this protects the muscle against injury.

Hold the stretch long enough to allow the stretch reflex to diminish and the lengthening reaction to occur.

To learn more about which stretches affect different parts of the body, I suggest you ask a personal trainer, or you can also find a lot of good information online.

No matter what type of stretch you do, never bounce as you do it. Don't hold your breath during the stretch. Stretches should be relaxed; increase the stretch gradually, but never to the point of pain. Take slow, relaxed breaths while stretching; exhale during the maximum points of the stretch. The breaths will help you feel more release of tension.

BALANCE

Balance is an aspect of fitness that closely relates to your long-term health. It needs to worked on just as you do for your core strength and flexibility. Balance involves three different systems within the body. The first system is in your inner ear. The inner ear has a compartment with special cells that tell the body about its position or motion. The second system is your visual system, which tells your brain about your position or motion based on what you see. The third system is called proprioception, meaning your own awareness of your body's movements.

Proprioception is your unconscious ability to know where you are in space without looking—it's how you can touch type or put food in your mouth without seeing what you're doing. Feedback from receptors in your muscles, tendons, and joints tell you where in space they actually are at the moment. Raise your hand above your head, but don't look at it. You can tell where it is without looking—proprioception in action.

If there's a weak link in the chain of the three systems, then your balance can be affected. The systems overlap to minimize any problems. For instance, if you couldn't tell where your hand was when you raised it, you would have instinctively looked at it to solve the problem. Your body uses these systems without the need for you to have to think about it. Often, you only notice a lack of balance when one system is shut down. For example, you may feel perfectly balanced in the shower, but if you close your eyes to rinse shampoo out of your hair, you may feel a little off balance. This is because the visual stimuli has been taken away, exposing a weakness in the three-pronged system.

As we get older, maintaining good balance becomes vital for continuing to do our daily activities with ease. With good balance, carrying something up dimly lit stairs, hiking on a rocky path, or just playing in the yard with your kids or grandkids will be easier and more carefree. As we get even older, good balance and movement are vital to avoid falls and continue to live independently. Fortunately, balance can be trained and improved at any age.

You need all three systems for good balance, but the only one you can actually improve through your exercise program is proprioception. Core training, strength training (particularly with free weights, because you control the range of motion), and, for that matter, almost any form of exercise can help. The difference is in how specific these activities are for maintaining and improving balance. As with any exercise, you want to get the most benefit for the time spent.

Some of the most simple and effective balance exercises can be done virtually anywhere in a matter of one or two minutes. You can make them part of your regular workout, or you can do them at any time when you have an idle moment during the day. You could do a balance exercise while waiting for your computer to boot up or for the coffee to brew, or during a commercial break while watching TV.

Any one of these three exercises is valuable. Switch them around or rotate them for even more benefit.

The first balance exercise is simply standing on one leg while you bend the other leg at the knee and lift it. It's OK to hold on to a table or chair back or touch the wall for balance if you need to. Start by doing each leg for 10 seconds—longer if you can. The goal is to stand for a total of one minute on each leg, either by adding short periods together or by working up to one full minute per leg at a time. I have an 84-year-old patient who at first could only do a few seconds while holding on to the wall. He followed the two-minute plan. Within six months he could balance while counting to a hundred without holding on to anything!

The second exercise is walking heel to toe along a straight line, as if you were walking on a tightrope. You've probably seen this on TV shows when police stop someone suspected of driving while intoxicated—it requires some concentration. Touch a wall for balance if you need to; and it's OK to put your arms out to the side. Practice until you can do this steadily for up to one minute.

The third exercise is standing on one leg while extending the other. Stand sideways next to a wall so you can support yourself if needed. Stand on one leg and extend the other leg out in front of you, so that your heel is six to 12 inches off the floor. Keep the extended leg straight and your toes pointed upward at about a 30-degree angle. Again, the goal is one minute total per leg, either in additive increments or all at once if you can.

You can do these exercises during idle time at home or even at work, or you can take a couple minutes at the gym. You can also try doing them on equipment such as wobble boards (also called balance boards), balance beams on the ground, or even a trampoline if you feel like mixing things up. Regardless of how or where you do it, you will get a big return on your time.

YOGA AND TAI CHI

Yoga and tai chi are two approaches that can be a valuable part of core, flexibility, and balance training. Both approaches are mind-body practices that use slow, gentle, low-impact exercise to build strength and improve balance.

YOGA

Yoga is a broad term for a combination of meditation and exercise meant to improve your flexibility, strength, and balance while also lowering stress—in yoga, the mind and body are one. Yoga originated thousands of years ago in India. Today, it's popular around the world in many different styles, including some, such as ashtanga yoga or hot yoga, that are very challenging. For improving balance, getting a low-impact workout, and relieving stress, I suggest the gentler form known as hatha yoga. In hatha yoga, the focus is on asanas, or yoga poses. While some asanas are very difficult, hatha yoga as it's usually taught incorporates simple poses that are easy to learn.

Yoga classes in a gym setting tend to focus on the physical aspects, with less attention to breathing and meditation. A private studio class may include more of the spiritual side of yoga, though it might be even more physically challenging. Your yoga class should have the feel and the level of intensity you're looking for. Ask questions and observe or take a class before deciding to sign up.

The yoga instructor is a key element to learning the asanas and having an enjoyable experience. Find a skilled and knowledgeable instructor who can understand your level of fitness and any limitations you have and help you get started safely. Look for someone who is also a good match for your needs and personality.

When you go to yoga class, try to have an empty stomach, meaning you haven't eaten for at least 90 minutes. Mental focus, concentration, and quiet meditation are part of yoga classes that primarily focus on the physical, so leave your cell phone in the locker room and plan to stay the full length of the class. Wear comfortable clothing as you would for other athletic activities; avoid any attire that's constricting. You don't need to worry about athletic shoes because you won't wear them (or your socks) during class.

Yoga uses some props to help you with the poses. The main prop is a yoga mat to provide some cushioning on the floor. (If you haven't decided if yoga is for you, ask the instructor about borrowing or renting a mat before you buy one.) Other props include folded blankets, towels, or foam blocks to support part of your body and straps, which are used to reach parts of your body you normally couldn't touch. For instance, you might wrap a strap around your foot if you can't reach your toes with your fingers.

In the yoga studio, position yourself on your mat facing the front of the room. Leave enough room between your neighbors so you have space to stretch out your arms and legs in the poses. Before the class starts, do some gentle stretching, or sit quietly and get mentally ready. Once class starts, do the poses as well as you can, following the form the instructor demonstrates. If you need to, stop and rest until you are ready to move back into the poses. If a movement causes pain or cramping, ease up. Yoga is supposed to make you feel better, not worse. Your instructor may gently touch you to help you do the pose with better form, but she shouldn't adjust you or force you into a position.

The class ends with savasana, a short meditation period when you can lie on your back, relax, and take in what you just did in class. Savasana is just as important as the poses. If you really must leave class early, tell the instructor beforehand and still do a short savasana before leaving.

When you begin your yoga practice, instruction is almost a necessity. As you become more proficient, you might find that a yoga mat in a quiet place in your home is a good alternative or addition to class. You can find many good yoga videos online— follow along or use them to get ideas for poses to incorporate into your home practice.

TAI CHI

Tai chi is an ancient mind-body practice that originated in China. Today, this mixture of physical and mental disciplines is very popular in the rest of the world as well. Tai chi has been described as "moving meditation." It's self-paced, gentle, and noncompetitive. Tai chi movements are performed in a slow but flowing pattern without pausing. There's no impact or jumping.

In the West, tai chi is usually taught as a series of 20 basic movements. They're easy to learn, emphasize balance and flow, and don't involve any stress on the joints. To learn tai chi, look for a qualified instructor, either at your gym or at a private studio—some martial arts schools also offer tai chi classes. No particular equipment is required; just wear comfortable clothing that doesn't hinder your movement. Once you know the tai chi forms, you can practice them just about anywhere. You may find it a nice change of pace from your regular aerobic routine.

CHAPTER 12
NUTRIENT TIMING

A S THE SAYING GOES, sometimes it's all in the timing. You can accomplish the lion's share of your fitness goals by following the YOU+ program as already described, but nutrient timing will take you to another level. You'll break through plateaus in your weight control, level of exercise capacity, and strength. Advances in these three areas improve insulin efficiency and lessen the risk of diseases that rob you of energy as well as shorten the length and quality of your life. By maximizing the improvements you've already made, you'll reap even greater benefits.

For many, following the path of fitness is like something I saw recently at the mall. It was late, and my wife and I had just seen a movie. As we were leaving the theater, we came out to an area in front of some escalators. As you might expect, this was the hangout spot for young teens waiting for their parents to pick them up. What they were doing to entertain themselves is what struck me. It was quite simple. They were trying to climb up the down escalator or down the up escalator. Isn't that what accomplishing your fitness regimen can feel like? You make an effort and achieve some improvements, but you don't always get as far as you want. You make a little progress or at least hold steady, but as soon as you let up a little, the escalator moves you in the wrong direction. What we need to do is to slow the escalator down. You'll still have to make an effort to see progress, but reaching the end of the escalator will now become that much more attainable.

The key factors for achieving greater progress through nutrient timing are what you do before and immediately after exercising. This is an area where nutrition and nutritional supplements play a vital role. As with the earlier discussion of food and dietary supplements (check back to section 2 on nutrition), the foods and supplements I'll discuss here aren't strange or unusual. They're found naturally in a typical diet; you eat them all the time. The beneficial effect on your fitness comes from consuming them at the right time and in the right amounts for maximum impact on your fitness.

PRE-EXERCISE MEAL

What you eat for your pre-workout meal is not going to result in marked improvements. The timing strategy that comes with your workout is where the improvements arise. Your pre-exercise meals or drinks, however, could hinder your results if not done properly.

Go to any gym and you'll see someone downing a sugar-laden sports drink or energy drink before working out. Although the caffeine in an energy drink can help performance, the overall effect of swallowing down a sugary drink right before exercise is almost always detrimental. The belief is that the sugar in the drink will "feed the muscles" and contribute to having enough energy for the workout. This simply isn't true.

In Chapter 9 on aerobic exercise, we touched on how energy is produced by your cells during exercise. You might remember that the body uses ATP for energy, and that ATP can be made from pathways that use glucose, protein, or fat. During the first 60 minutes, or even up to the first 90 minutes of exercise, your body uses glycogen, a form of glucose that's stored in your muscles. When you're doing aerobic exercise, your body draws on the glycogen in your muscles to make ATP for energy. Unless you plan to work out for longer than 60 to 90 minutes, your body already has enough stored glucose to power your exercise. So, all the sugar in that sports drink you just threw down is nothing but extra calories, which will be stored later as fat. No matter how many calories you burn with your exercise, you will lower the net amount by the sugar calories you just drank.

The same argument can be made for your weight-lifting workouts. Your body already has enough glucose stored as glycogen to take care of your energy needs. You don't need to add more from food or drink right before you exercise. For instance, even after six sets of ten repetitions working a particular muscle, you still have about 60 percent of that muscle's glycogen supply left.

Taking in sugar from something like a sports drink before exercise has another downside. When you consume sugar, your insulin levels rise. This is not what you want at this stage of your workout. The rise in insulin can actually cause your blood sugar level to drop during exercise; it may go down to a level lower than it would have without the sugar intake. This can lead to lower exercise capacity because when your blood sugar is low, you just don't feel like doing what you might normally do.

Some argue that taking in sugary carbohydrates right before exercise can be beneficial because it can lower the rise in your cortisol level. This stress hormone can go up with exercise. This is true, but the cortisol rise naturally becomes smaller when you exercise regularly. You don't need to take in the extra sugar.

WHEN TO EAT

Research suggests that the optimal time to eat before exercise is from one to three hours before. I personally find that I do best at the longer end of this range. If you exercise first thing in the morning, it's OK to skip eating before your workout if doing so makes you feel uncomfortable—having food in your stomach from eating right before exercise can cause stomach discomfort, bloating, and sluggishness for some. Even after fasting overnight while you were asleep, you'll still have enough glucose stored as glycogen to power you through your workout. If you exercise later in the day or in the evening, the meal ratio structure outlined in Chapter 5 will give you enough energy and nutrients for optimal exercise if you time your meal for that one- to three-hour pre-exercise window.

The optimal pre-workout meal consists of slow-digesting carbohydrates, such as whole grains, and protein. This combination best keeps your blood sugar and insulin at appropriate levels and allows you to complete your regimen without interference from other factors.

BUILDING BLOCKS

The key to optimal nutrient timing lies in amino acids, the building blocks of protein. Each of the 20 amino acids that are the backbone of protein structure in the human body has different characteristics. Taking advantage of these characteristics is the goal of the YOU+ supplementation strategy.

When I say that amino acids are the building blocks of protein, I mean that quite literally. Put simply, proteins are amino acids strung together in different sequences and formations. The 20 amino acids that are so important for making the proteins in your body are an integral part of the genetic code. Just as Morse code has dots and dashes to signify letters, our DNA has groupings known as codons that represent each of the 20 amino acids. By translating the codons (the body's version of the Morse code's dots and dashes), the DNA in your cells tells the body what protein structures (muscle, hormones, enzymes, and others) to make.

Each amino acid is different. Some can be manufactured within the body, but others can't be made—you have to eat them. Nine of the 20 amino acids must be supplied by your diet. These nine amino acids are called essential amino acids for that reason: it is essential that you get them from your food. This is the same distinction we make with essential fatty acids—they're essential because your body can't make them, so they have to be part of your diet.

EATING YOUR AMINOS

The nine essential amino acids are easily found in everyday foods. Foods that have all the essential amino acids in adequate amounts are known as complete. This generally applies to all animal proteins, including meat, fish, eggs, and dairy.

Most plant foods are incomplete, meaning that they lack sufficient amounts of one or more of the nine essential amino acids. This doesn't mean that plant foods are less healthy. It simply means that to meet your amino acid needs, you need to combine different plant foods. For example, corn is low in lysine but high in methionine and cysteine. Beans are high in lysine and low in methionine and cysteine. By combining both incomplete proteins, you get enough of all the essential amino acids for good health, even if you don't eat them all at a single meal. If you don't eat animal foods, the best way to be sure of getting enough of all the essential amino acids is to eat a wide variety of foods.

Some plant products are complete proteins. Soy is the most common. Amaranth and quinoa are grain-like seeds from Central and South America. Buckwheat, also known as kasha or soba (in Japanese cooking), is another good choice.

If you follow the YOU+ eating plan outlined in Chapter 5, you'll get all the complete protein you need from your regular meals. Taking amino acid supplements, however, can give you an indispensable workout advantage through the timing, speed, ratio, amount, and efficiency of delivery. Supplementing greatly increases how quickly and efficiently you can get the appropriate amounts of the necessary nutrients to where you need them, and at the right time. Three sources of amino acids are particularly valuable for building your fitness: branched chain amino acids (BCAAs), glutamine, and whey protein.

BRANCHED CHAIN AMINO ACIDS

The branched chain amino acids (BCAAs) are three of the nine essential amino acids we were just discussing. Branched chain refers to the shape of the amino acids leucine, isoleucine, and valine. The BCAAs have been extensively studied in people of all ages. The bottom line is that their correct use in supplements can lead to reduced fat mass and optimization of lean muscle mass. The most important BCAA for fat loss and muscle mass seems to be leucine, but many of the studies involve all three of the BCAAs or even all of the essential amino acids, which include the BCAAs.

Although the BCAAs can help you shed fat and optimize muscle, I need to emphasize that they are not remotely related to steroids or other hormones. They are simply a natural component of many foods. For woman, BCAAs will help you achieve a toned, healthy, feminine physique. For men, they will help you achieve a leaner, more defined, athletic physique. For both men and woman, this can lead to a more active, fit, and healthy life.

We know from plenty of studies that the body uses more BCAAs during exercise. Based on this observation, researchers wondered if providing BCAAs to the body in the right amount at the correct time could improve muscle growth. In fact, this turns out to be true. Multiple studies show that those who have higher levels of BCAAs at the correct time and concentration make more muscle protein during the recovery period just after exercise. This leads to a cascade of positive changes that will eventually improve insulin efficiency, reduce insulin resistance, and give you all of the associated benefits.

The increase in protein synthesis from BCAA supplementation can be in the order of 33 percent. This is true even for older adults, although they may need to take more BCAAs to achieve the same effect. This is a cause of considerable optimism because it shows we can overcome many of the negative effects of aging, despite the naturally occurring drop in hormone levels.

Studies also suggest that getting BCAAs at the right time and concentration can also help decrease your amount of abdominal fat over time. It's abdominal fat that produces many of the damaging substances in the ongoing struggle between the two opposing forces of breakdown and repair. Decreasing abdominal fat will also improve your insulin efficiency.

BCAAs also help limit muscle damage and breakdown during exercise. We want some muscle breakdown during exercise because it's the repair of the breakdown that leads to gains in fitness. The BCAAs enable the repair process, allowing for maximum gains in fitness without the downside of breakdown. A study in the *Journal of Nutrition* showed that supplementation with BCAAs lowers the amount of muscle soreness and fatigue that can occur for a few days after exercise. Other studies have found lower levels of the biochemical markers of muscle breakdown, supporting the idea that BCAAs offer a fitness advantage.

People who take BCAA supplements take longer to fatigue during exercise, both mentally and physically. A recent study showed that exercisers who supplemented with BCAAs rated their perceived exertion (using a scale similar to the Willey exertion scale) as lower than those who didn't take the supplement. This suggests that BCAAs can help you do more without feeling that it's more effort. A study in the *Journal of Sports Medicine and Physical Fitness* reported that those who took the branched chain amino acids took 17 percent longer to feel tired when they started their exercise while already in a fatigued state.

GLUTAMINE

The next item on our supplement list is glutamine, another amino acid. Glutamine isn't an essential amino acid. Instead, it's conditionally essential, which simply means that most of the time, your body can make all it needs. Under certain conditions, however, your body can't make enough of it. During these times, glutamine becomes essential, and you need to get it from your diet or supplements.

Glutamine is the most abundant amino acid in muscle. It's a primary fuel source for the immune system and for our digestive tract. The effects of glutamine have been most closely studied in patients who are very ill in an intensive care unit. For these patients, intravenous glutamine can be valuable for preventing muscle wasting and boosting the immune system.

The temporary stress of exercise is clearly not in the same league as the stress of being in intensive care, but exercise can still make glutamine conditionally essential.

Glutamine is a valuable supplement for helping to heal your intestines if they've been damaged by increased gut permeability and the inflammation it causes (check back to Chapter 3). In fact, I feel glutamine is so important for your overall health that

I recommend it as a daily supplement—I'll explain more about that later in this chapter.

I believe glutamine has an additional role in helping you meet your fitness goals. Researchers studying very sick patients found that glutamine limited muscle wasting; they thought that glutamine might therefore help limit muscle loss and damage from exercise, much as branched chain amino acids do. The case for this isn't very strong, however glutamine does appear to help in the recovery from exercise. Supplements of glutamine help the muscles rebuild their levels of glycogen, or stored glucose, back to their maximum level. Eating carbohydrates will also restore glycogen, but glutamine can do it *without* the extra calories.

Glutamine's ability to restore glycogen levels may also enhance insulin efficiency, which means your body needs to produce less insulin. In one study, consuming glutamine along with a carbohydrate increased the rate of glucose disposal by 25 percent two hours after exercise. In this same study, glutamine on its own was shown to enhance glycogen replacement as much as a glucose supplement did. More evidence of glutamine's potential ability to lower insulin resistance came from a study of people with diabetes. Those who took glutamine along with their insulin had more instances of their blood sugar dropping low overnight, indicating that the glutamine enhanced their sensitivity to insulin.

Another advantage of glutamine is its role in fueling the immune system. When glutamine levels are low, the immune system doesn't function optimally. In theory, taking glutamine when your levels are lower, such as after exercise, might keep you from getting sick as often. The theory may well be true— studies have found lower rates of infections in those who took glutamine after exercise.

Glutamine levels can also be affected by the BCAAs. Having plenty of branched chain amino acids in your system appears to keep glutamine levels higher after exercise, which is yet another desirable effect. Even if you use BCAA supplements, however, glutamine supplements are important.

In general, I recommend 5 grams of supplemental glutamine daily, whether or not you work out that day. Take the supplemental glutamine whenever it's convenient for you. It comes as a tasteless powder than can easily be mixed into anything. On a workout day, you'll be getting some extra glutamine from your post-workout whey shake (I'll explain more about that later in this chapter), but it's still important to get that extra 5 grams beyond what's in the shake.

WHEY PROTEIN

Whey protein is the third element in the YOU+ nutrient timing strategy. Whey protein is one of the constituents of milk. Remember the nursery rhyme that goes, "Little Miss Muffet sat on a tuffet, eating her curds and whey"? When milk is curdled to make cheese or yogurt, whey is the watery liquid left behind. To make whey protein supplements, the liquid is dried into a powder.

The protein in the whey contains all nine essential amino acids, but it's especially rich in the BCAAs leucine, isoleucine, and valine. In fact, just over 25 percent of the content of whey protein is BCAAs—and almost 20 percent of whey protein is glutamine. In addition, the amino acid profile and the proportion of amino acids in whey protein are very similar to that of skeletal muscle. Whey protein is valuable as a supplement for all of these reasons alone, but it also has some other wonderful properties that, when used properly, can be very useful for meeting your fitness and health goals.

The first of these properties is whey protein's speed of absorption and action in the bloodstream. It is tailor-made for use in a nutrient timing strategy because we can plan exactly how much to take and know precisely when it will start working. Amino acids from whey protein begin to appear in the bloodstream about 20 minutes after you ingest them. They don't stay there long—they're usually fully taken up and used by your body within 90 minutes. The timing and change in the concentration of amino acids is important for stimulating protein synthesis. By concentrating quickly in the blood, whey protein accomplishes this quite nicely. Because of whey protein's high concentration of quickly absorbed BCAAs, the raw materials you need to stimulate protein synthesis will be present just when you need them.

Whey protein also tends to promote greater leanness. You might expect this, because whey protein is high in BCAAs, and we know BCAAs promote leanness, but there's actually more to this benefit. Whey protein is a potent stimulator of the gastrointestinal hormones called incretins (check back to Chapter 1). Incretins are helpful for weight control in several ways, including improving insulin efficiency and making you feel full more quickly. In studies, the subjects who took whey protein tended to eat less in subsequent meals.

Whey may also help promote leanness by changing gene expression in the muscle. We talked earlier about how diet and exercise can change which genes are activated and which genes are deactivated, allowing you some control over your genetic destiny. A study in the *Journal of Nutrigenetics and Nutrigenomics* found that whey protein beneficially altered the expression of genes in skeletal muscle that would be expected to promote leanness.

Many of my patients have had success with weight loss by having a whey protein shake for breakfast and/or lunch. The shake cuts their appetite while still providing good nutrition. If achieving your desired weight is a primary goal, try whey shakes.

In addition to these considerable benefits, whey can be a potent antioxidant. It helps increase your level of glutathione, your body's most abundant natural antioxidant. Whey protein is an excellent good source of the amino acid cysteine, which your body needs to make glutathione and which is sometimes in short supply in your body. Studies have shown that people who take a whey-based supplement have higher levels of glutathione in their system.

THE BIOLOGICAL VALUE OF WHEY PROTEIN

Your body uses whey protein very efficiently. To know exactly how efficiently, we can measure what percentage of the protein you ingest actually gets utilized by your body using a unit known as the biological value (BV). This term is often thrown around inaccurately or misleadingly by nutritional supplement marketers. That's because biological value can be looked at in two different ways.

One approach to biological value is the basic way, which looks at the simple percentage of a protein used by the body. It stands to reason that your body can't use more than 100 percent of a protein, so this approach is pretty straightforward and logical. The second approach however, looks at the biological value of a protein in comparison to the protein in an egg. Because eggs contain all the essential amino acids in about the same proportions your body needs, they're considered the gold standard for comparing and rating other protein sources. Egg protein is given a score of 100, and all other proteins are rated based on that. In terms of traditional biological value, egg protein is outstanding at around 94 percent utilization. However, some proteins rank even higher for their BV. They have a BV score higher than 100 because they're being compared to egg protein, not on their own absolute BV percentage.

Whey protein is one of those superior proteins. Its biological value on this comparative scale is 104. So, a protein can have a score higher than 100. The calculation has just been made differently. No matter how you look at it, whey is a fabulous protein source.

THE STRATEGY

Now you know the reasoning behind BCAA, glutamine, and whey protein supplements. Next comes knowing when and how to use them.

BCAA SUPPLEMENTATION BEFORE EXERCISE

BCAA supplements should be taken just before you start your workout. The supplements aren't that easy to find in a local health-food store or vitamin shop; you may need to order them online from a reliable supplier. I recommend taking them in capsule form because they have a very bitter taste. Some manufacturers are now making flavored BCAA powders; they're certainly worth trying. Unfortunately, many BCAA supplements also include other ingredients that are unnecessary and just make the supplements more expensive. Look for a product that contains only the BCAAs and contains at least 50 percent leucine.

A few minutes before you start your exercise, take a total of 3 to 5 grams (3,000 to 5,000 milligrams) of BCAAs. If you're over age 50, aim for the higher end of the range. Swallow them down with plain water. As long as you haven't eaten for 90 minutes before you start, the aminos will be fully absorbed into your system quickly enough to have a beneficial effect on your muscles, fat burning, and perceived exertion during your exercise session. Take the BCAAs no matter what type of exercise—aerobic or resistance—you're doing that day.

WHEY PROTEIN AFTER EXERCISE

What supplements you take after exercise depends on what type of exercise you did. I divide the type of exercise into three different categories. The first category is a normal cardio session of up to 30 minutes. The second category is a resistance or strength-training workout, regardless of whether or not you included any aerobic exercise in the same workout. The third is aerobic activity that includes an element of resistance exercise, such as swimming, stationary bike with resistance, or a rowing machine for 30 minutes or more, or a cardio session that lasts for 60 minutes or more, regardless of the type of exercise you do.

For the first category, a standard aerobic session, you don't need to take any supplements afterward. The BCAAs you took before starting will accomplish what you need for protein synthesis and recovery.

For both the second and third category workouts, which put different demands on your muscles, your supplements after exercise should be timed to provide optimal protein synthesis and restoration of glycogen. The best way to accomplish this is by taking whey protein right after you have finished your workout. To be crystal clear on this point, that means you need to take your whey protein immediately after you complete your workout. Whey protein gives you a good supply of BCAAs and glutamine, so it's perfect to support recovery, repair, and fat loss.

I recommend that you take 20 to 25 grams of whey protein powder mixed with around 10 grams of carbohydrate from a rapidly absorbing source, such as Gatorade powder. Mix the powders together with about 12 ounces of water in a shaker cup. I usually put a 20- to 25-gram scoop of whey protein powder (I like the vanilla ice cream flavor) in my shaker cup, along with the 10 grams of powdered Gatorade. I throw this in my gym bag along with the bottle of BCAAs. I take my BCAAs before I start. When I'm finished with my workout, I simply go to the water fountain, add water to the whey protein/Gatorade mix, shake it up, and drink it down.

Be sure to take your post-workout supplements immediately after your session. The time window for achieving the desired response is limited. If you don't take the supplements within 60 minutes of finishing your workout, much of the potential benefit will be lost. In fact, if you get past two hours after exercise, the tables will turn on you. Not only have you missed your window, but your muscles will become resistant to the effects. This is the main reason the rapid absorption speed of whey protein is so important. Other proteins or solid food just won't be absorbed in time to be as helpful.

I recommend mixing your whey powder with around 10 grams of a rapidly absorbed carbohydrate, such as a sports drink powder. This adds only 40 calories to the drink, but the return on the calorie investment is worthwhile. When the carbohydrate combines with the glutamine in the whey protein, it restores the glycogen supply of your muscles quickly. By restoring the glycogen supply, your body recovers more quickly, is more prepared for the next workout, and may be less prone to injury and overtraining. In addition, adding a carbohydrate to a whey protein mixture after exercise may give a further boost to protein synthesis.

SLEEP, STRESS, AND MOTIVATION

CHAPTER 13
SLEEP

S LEEP IS AN INTEGRAL component of fitness, yet a good night's sleep is an elusive goal for many. Sleep's impact on health and fitness is immense. Sleep, or the lack of it, affects both our quality of life and the frequency of health problems.

The quality of life issue is obvious. Whether it's that dreadful feeling of having to crawl out of bed for a morning obligation when you're still dead tired, or fighting to stay awake in a meeting or while driving home, we all know that lack of sleep takes the steam out of our day. Without adequate sleep, we can be crabby, ill-tempered, and run-down. Studies confirm that we don't perform as well on either mental or physical tasks when we are sleep deprived. Improving the quality of your sleep can make you feel better and happier. That's reason enough to explore how to improve your sleep. However, the story only begins there.

SLEEP AND WEIGHT GAIN

Lack of sleep and weight gain aren't obviously connected, but the link is very real. Only recently, however, have we started to understand why sleep and weight are connected. To take just one good study, the health statistics division of the Centers for

Disease Control and Prevention (CDC) surveyed 87,000 people between 2004 and 2006. They found that 33 percent of people who slept less than six hours a night were obese, but only 22 percent of "normal sleepers" (seven to eight hours a night) were obese. The study convincingly showed that sleep duration was indeed associated with obesity in those who slept less than six hours a night. Another interesting study of 384,541 people, published in BMC Public Health in 2011, showed that there was a linear relationship between the number of nights in the last 30 days that subjects reported sleep difficulties and their body mass index. In other words, the more nights with sleep difficulties, the higher the body mass index—another way of saying that people who consistently sleep poorly or not enough tend to be overweight.

Why poor sleeping is related to weight gain isn't completely understood, but we have some pretty good ideas. If you don't get enough sleep, you may experience fluctuations in the hormonal signals your body uses to tell you if you're hungry or full. We touched on this concept back in Chapter 1, in the explanation of how gastrointestinal hormones and a higher-protein diet make us feel full for longer. When it comes to sleep, two of the same appetite signals are affected. If you're short on sleep, your production of the hunger hormone ghrelin increases, while your production of feel-full hormone leptin decreases. When you combine the imbalanced appetite hormones caused by lack of sleep with the way being tired lowers your willpower, then add in how readily available food is everywhere you go, the connection between sleep and weight gain becomes clear. In addition, when the ghrelin and leptin signals are impaired by lack of sleep, you tend to crave high-calorie, high-sugar foods, therefore adding to the problem. The good news is that when the test subjects got adequate sleep, the hormonal imbalances disappeared. If this situation sounds familiar to you, take heart—you can fix it.

SLEEP AND MEDICAL PROBLEMS

Lack of adequate sleep is associated with an increased risk of dying prematurely, greater insulin resistance, high blood pressure, heart disease, diabetes, change in hormone levels, and depression. The risk of death from inadequate sleep has been known for some time. In the 1980s, a study that followed 1.1 million people reported on the risk of death as it related to sleep duration. This study found that people who slept six hours or less nightly had a significantly higher risk of dying during the follow-up period of the study. Those who slept five hours or less were even worse off.

In the Nurses' Health Study, over 71,000 female health professionals were followed for their risk of coronary heart disease as it related to their sleep duration. Even after adjusting for multiple factors, including weight and smoking, the women who slept six hours or less nightly had a higher risk of coronary heart disease. As in the mortality study, getting less than five hours of sleep a night increased the risk even further. A study published in the journal *Sleep* found that those who slept less than six hours nightly had a 23 percent higher risk for heart disease even after controlling for other variables. This number jumped to a 79 percent higher risk if the sleep was also of poor quality.

A study in the journal *Cancer* revealed that those sleeping less than six hours nightly had an almost 50 percent increase in colorectal adenomas, a type of polyp that can lead to colon cancer. Other studies have shown that men who don't sleep well are up to twice as likely to develop prostate cancer as those who do sleep well.

Studies that look at insulin resistance as it relates to sleep duration have found remarkably similar results. Lack of insulin efficiency is increased by sleep deprivation. If you don't sleep enough, your body needs more insulin than it should to get the job done; hence, your insulin levels are higher than they need to be (check back to Chapter 1 for more on insulin efficiency). Sleeping just five hours every night, for a period as short as one week has been shown to significantly increase insulin resistance. You don't have to be that severely sleep deprived for your insulin resistance to go up. It will happen even if you just sleep for less time than is usual for you over a period of a couple weeks. And it will happen even if you're a lean young adult, which only shows that optimizing your insulin efficiency is important for everyone.

SLEEP TYPES AND FRAGMENTATION

In order to improve your sleep, it's first helpful to understand a little more about it, including what's within the normal range.

Sleep is your body's time for rest and restoration. Even though you're not moving around while you're asleep, your brain and body are actually still quite active. In fact, your brain is almost as active when you're asleep as when you're awake. Sleep itself is an active state—you pass through a number of sleep stages in the course of a night. The stages fall into two basic stages: rapid eye movement (REM) sleep and non-rapid eye movement (NREM) sleep. During NREM sleep, you normally pass through four different stages. As you sleep, you cycle through the REM and NREM stages; each cycle takes roughly 90 minutes.

When you first fall asleep, you move into NREM sleep. You typically pass through four stages of this type of sleep over the next 90 minutes or so; each stage lasts anywhere from 5 to 20 minutes. In stage 1, you are lightly asleep and can easily be awakened—this stage usually lasts for about 5 to 10 minutes. From there, you move into stage 2 sleep. You're still lightly asleep and can easily be woken up, but now your heart beats more slowly, and your body temperature drops a bit as your body prepares to go into deeper sleep. During stage 3 sleep, you are deeply asleep and hard to wake; from this stage, you move into stage 4 sleep, which is even deeper. While you are in stages 3 and 4, your body is in peak repair mode. This is when you repair and rebuild all parts of your body, including your muscles and your immune system. Because of this, stages 3 and 4 are often referred to as restorative sleep.

After you've been through a full cycle of NREM sleep, you move into a period of REM sleep. During REM sleep, you have the rapid eye movements behind closed lids that are characteristic of this stage; during at least some of your REM sleep, you have dreams. Your first REM stage usually lasts only about 10 minutes. With each additional sleep cycle, the REM stage gets longer; your last REM stage could last up to an hour. That's why you're more likely to remember dreams in the morning.

At the beginning of your sleep time, you spend more time in NREM sleep. Overall, it's the longest part of your sleep time, making up approximately 75 percent of your total sleep time as a young adult. Older adults spend less time in NREM sleep.

When the normal sleep cycle is interrupted for some reason (caring for a sick child, for example, or feeling worried or ill yourself), you experience sleep fragmentation, and this may cause you to not feel well rested in the morning. In fact, sleep fragmentation is the most common cause of daytime sleepiness.

A common misconception is that sleep is only normal if you sleep through the night for eight hours without waking. As the night goes on and you pass through the sleep cycles, it's normal to wake up for a short period between cycles. As this type of awakening is part of the natural cycle, it's not the same as sleep fragmentation, which affects the quality of your sleep. Sometimes, worrying about this phenomenon causes more problems than the lack of sleep itself!

Everyone is different when it comes to sleep. Our need for sleep may change, depending on work patterns, lifestyle, and age. Older people, for example, tend to sleep less, although the amount of sleep needed doesn't appear to decrease as we age; if they wake up during the night, they may stay awake for longer. We also know that older people spend less time in the deeper stages of sleep (stages 3 and 4). Fit seniors, however, often sleep as well as their younger counterparts. Better sleep probably also leads to improved cognition in seniors.

HOW MUCH SLEEP DO YOU NEED?

We know from many studies, such as the ones mentioned above, that consistently getting less than six hours of sleep a night can negatively affect your health in a variety of different ways. However, preventing disease and functioning at your peak level are two very different things when it comes to sleep. Most experts recommend that the average adult get seven to nine hours of sleep per night for optimal health. Individuals can vary quite a bit in their sleep needs. Some people feel fine on just six hours of sleep, while others need at least eight. There's no formula for how much sleep to get, but it's pretty clear that sleeping less than six hours a night increases your risk of disease and being overweight. The amount of sleep that makes you feel best is probably the amount you need.

Of course, not everyone can hope to have a great night's sleep every night. Life is complex, and situations will always arise where you lose sleep or are not able to rest as much as you need or want. If you need to do shift work, for instance, your sleep pattern will probably be somewhat disrupted or fragmented. This is where the concept of the sleep bank comes in. When you get less than sleep than you need, you develop a sleep debt. You'll make a withdrawal from your sleep bank. The good news is that you can pay back your sleep debt or make a deposit to the sleep bank by getting some extra sleep on subsequent nights. That lets your body catch up on the sleep it needs. If you owe sleep to your sleep bank, your body will spend more time in the deeper stages 3 and 4 of sleep to make up for the sleep debt. Catching up takes some time, however, so try not to burn the candle at both ends too often. Studies have shown that extra sleep over the weekend isn't usually quite enough to fully recover from a sleep-deprived workweek.

Another useful way to repay your sleep debt is to have a short nap in the afternoon. Napping takes advantage of your body's circadian rhythm, or its natural cycle of sleeping and waking. Your circadian rhythm is connected to your brain in complex ways; it's controlled in large part by exposure to light and dark. Although your body's greatest drive for sleep is at night, your circadian rhythm also drives you toward a natural desire for some sleep in the afternoon. Taking a short nap at this time is pretty natural. As long as it's not too long, a nap can help repay your sleep debt without impairing sleep at night. In many cultures, an afternoon nap, or siesta, is common. Finding half an hour for a siesta is hard for busy adults in our society, but if you can manage it, I recommend it if you need to repay sleep debt. You will probably find that you feel refreshed when you wake up. The extra alertness from your nap will last well into the evening.

SLEEP PROBLEMS

Unfortunately, getting adequate sleep is a big problem for a large segment of the population. Sometimes, lack of sleep is caused simply by not setting aside enough time for it. Certainly, we've built more and more tasks into our day, but the day still only has 24 hours. When we're done with all of our work, school, and family obligations for the day, we tend to just take a breather and relax, often with TV or video games or in front of a computer screen, rather than necessarily going to bed to get some well-earned sleep. In 1960, the average American got slightly more than eight hours of sleep per night. Now, the average has fallen to under seven hours per night. Although there are multiple other factors at play, it's probably not a coincidence that the rate of obesity has also skyrocketed during that time.

Sleep studies and surveys commonly show that at least one-third of the participants are experiencing insomnia, or a difficulty with sleeping. The problems are usually described as difficulty falling asleep, difficulty staying asleep, or restless sleep.

Insomnia generally falls into three types. Transient insomnia lasts only a few nights or less. It's usually caused by a stressful event, such as preparing for a big presentation or not feeling well. Short-term insomnia can last up to a month. It's frequently related to an emotionally disruptive event, such as the death of a loved one. The third and most debilitating category is chronic insomnia, which I define as sleep disruption that impairs your lifestyle for more than a month, even if you don't experience it every night.

COMMON CAUSES OF CHRONIC INSOMNIA

Stress is usually at the top of the list when it comes to causes of sleep problems. How many times have you had trouble falling asleep because something was on your mind and you couldn't shake it? Or how often have you awakened in the middle of the night ruminating over a situation? Chances are, if you go to bed stressed, you'll have some sort of problem sleeping—and the sleep you do get may be restless and fragmented.

A very common cause of sleep problems are habits that can make any of the other underlying sleep problems worse. As you will see, this is an area where many improvements can be made.

Substance abuse is another important cause of insomnia. The obvious frontrunner here is caffeine, which is a common cause of wakefulness, but that's only part of the story. Alcohol is probably the biggest cause of sleep disorders. Drinking alcohol may help you get to sleep, but once you're asleep, you may not stay that way. Alcohol-influenced sleep is likely to be fragmented and of poor quality. If you have problems sleeping, look carefully at your alcohol intake. I'm not suggesting you have to give up a glass of wine with dinner if you enjoy it, but be aware of how it could be affecting your sleep.

Smoking is obviously bad for you on every level—including sleep. Nicotine is a stimulant that can keep you awake. I genuinely hope that if you're reading this book, you're not currently a smoker. If you are and if you also experience insomnia, the link between the two is yet another good reason to give up smoking.

Sleep problems can also have medical causes. For example, certain medications, like beta blockers, often used to treat high blood pressure or heart problems, can cause insomnia. Sleep-disrupting side effects from drugs are a big contributor to why some older folks, who are more likely to be taking prescription drugs, don't sleep well. If you believe that a prescription drug is giving you insomnia, discuss it with your doctor. You might be able to switch to a different drug that won't keep you awake.

You might think you're relaxing when you watch TV or play a video game before going to sleep, but in fact, you could be keeping yourself from getting restful sleep. Electronic screens, including computers, tablets, and televisions, emit a lot of light in the invisible blue end of the color spectrum (ultraviolet light). Exposure to blue light has been shown to cause insomnia for many people. If you're having trouble sleeping, try to avoid looking at anything on a screen for a couple of hours before bedtime. You may discover that this is surprisingly helpful.

SLEEP APNEA

Obstructive sleep apnea is a condition where you frequently stop, or nearly stop, breathing while you're asleep. The pauses in your breathing can last for many seconds and can occur numerous times in an hour. Each time that your breathing becomes very shallow or stops, your sleep is disturbed, even if you don't wake up completely. As a result, your sleep is fragmented, and you feel tired during the day, even though you might have thought you slept well.

Obstructive sleep apnea happens because something is blocking your trachea, the airway that brings air into your lungs. The obstruction could be from your tongue, your tonsils, or your uvula; if you are overweight, it might be because you have a lot of fatty tissue in your throat area. People with sleep apnea usually snore very loudly, so often their bed partner is the first person to notice the symptoms. Your doctor should assess your sleep apnea to find out what's causing it. Weight loss can absolutely help, but many people need to use a special breathing apparatus to force air into their trachea while they sleep.

RESTLESS LEGS SYNDROME

Restless legs syndrome (RLS) is one of the more descriptive diagnoses in medicine. RLS is a disorder that makes your legs feel like they're gnawing, pulling, or creeping—and the sensation causes an overwhelming urge to move your legs to relieve the sensation. The symptoms of RLS usually occur at night, just when you're relaxing or in bed, and can get worse as the night goes on. If you have restless legs syndrome, you're likely unable to find a comfortable position, which keeps you from falling asleep and staying asleep. Most people with RLS don't get much restful sleep and have a lot of trouble with daytime sleepiness.

The cause of RLS is usually unknown for most people. It's sometimes related to diabetic peripheral neuropathy, so treating the
underlying diabetes may be helpful.

A BETTER NIGHT'S SLEEP

If insomnia is a problem for you, the best solution for getting
a better night's sleep may well be a form of behavioral therapy.
Good data support this approach. Studies have compared the
use of this simple method to prescription sleep medicines. Over
the long term, the behavioral approach compares favorably. One
study, published in the *Journal of the American Medical Association*, compared behavioral therapy to a common prescription
sleep medication. After six months, participants in the behavioral group spent more time in the more restorative NREM
stages 3 and 4 of sleep, spent less time awake at night, and had
greater total sleep time than the group taking the medication. In
other studies, behavioral therapy has been shown to help reduce
the time it takes to get to sleep or to go back to sleep after awakening at night by 30 minutes, and may increase the total time
spent asleep by up to an hour.

What makes behavioral therapy so effective is that it empha-
sizes how you have some control over sleep problems. And if
you have control over your sleep problems, you can change how
you respond to them. Behavioral therapy challenges you to stop
feeling powerless and defeated by insomnia. It teaches you how
to eliminate attitudes and approaches that aren't helpful and
teaches you better strategies for overcoming insomnia. Last but
not least, this type of therapy teaches you that worrying about
sleep may cause more problems than the insomnia itself.

Behavioral therapy is usually conducted by an instructor in
weekly sessions over a six-to eight-week period. This time-inten-
sive approach isn't always necessary. Many of my patients have

been successful by following the basic techniques of behavioral therapy on their own. This approach can easily be used by anyone.

The first step to changing sleep behavior is to address any obstacles to good sleep, such as not setting aside adequate time for sleep, medical problems, or substance abuse issues. Take charge of the things that you already know are having a negative impact on your sleep. This is easier to do if you understand sleep's importance for your fitness and how sleep may be a potent weapon for you in the battle of the bulge. You should probably know by now how much sleep you need each night to be productive the next day. Make it a priority to set aside appropriate time for the sleep you need. This step alone will enhance all of your other efforts.

The behavioral therapy approach relies on following some simple guidelines. Most of them are pretty easy; others will take a bit of commitment. The key here is to give the behavioral approach adequate time to work. If you've had sleep issues for several months or longer, be realistic. Your insomnia is not going to go away in just a few nights. Most people will need to follow the program for six to eight weeks to establish a regularly improved sleeping pattern, particularly if you have had chronic difficulties. Even if you don't think you have a sleep problem and just want to get a better night's sleep, the behavioral therapy approach will work for you as well.

BEHAVIORAL THERAPY APPROACH: STEP ONE

The first step in behavioral therapy for insomnia focuses on undoing habits that are counterproductive to achieving a good night's sleep.

- Only use your bedroom for sleep and sex. Your system needs to recognize that these are the *only* two things the bed is for. Watching television, working on your laptop, or other activities associated with wakefulness in the bedroom send the wrong signal. All of these activities create a pattern that reinforces the idea that it's normal to be awake in bed.

- Establish a relaxing pre-bed routine. This might include reading, listening to music, a warm bath, watching a TV show—essentially anything that doesn't require your brain to engage too fully and has nothing to do with stressful parts of your life. Use this time to get away from your worries so they don't resurface to wake you up later. In keeping with the first point, these activities should take place somewhere other than your bedroom. Repeating the same relaxing activity pattern over and over conditions your body to know that now it's time to get ready to sleep. Don't go to bed until you are ready to sleep or are already sleepy.

- About an hour before you want to go to sleep, dim the lights significantly. This helps trigger the circadian rhythms that influence sleep. This can be as simple as watching a TV show or listening to music in a darkened room, or dimming the lights to the lowest tolerable level for other activities.

- As simple as this sounds, invest in a comfortable mattress. This can be an investment that pays big rewards. Make sure your bedroom is comfortable in other ways as well: the right temperature, dark, and quiet.

BEHAVIORAL THERAPY APPROACH: STEP TWO

The second step in this type of therapy involves changing the way you approach sleep once you're actually in bed. This step is most helpful for those who have more chronic sleep difficulties. Step two is more challenging than step one. You need to be committed to following the program through. Stick with it— eventually, you will see results.

- Begin by staying in bed only for the number of hours you actually sleep at night. For instance, if you are in bed seven hours nightly but sleep only five of those hours, begin by scheduling only five hours to be in bed. Try to go to bed at about the same time every night. No matter when you go to bed, you must get out of bed after the time allotted—even if you're still tired. Do this no matter how much sleep you got. For example, if you went to bed at midnight and your allotted time was five hours, you would need to get up at 5 a.m.—no matter what. This is challenging. It's normal to experience some daytime drowsiness when you begin this process. For this reason, be cautious in your activities the following day, particularly if drowsiness could pose a danger.

- As you spend more time asleep each night, however, lengthen the amount of time you spend in bed. When you get to the point where you are asleep more than 80 or 90 percent of your time in bed, you can then increase your scheduled time in bed by 20 minutes. Following the example above, if you went to bed at midnight and stayed asleep for at least 80 percent of your allotted five hours, you would now get up at 5:20 a.m. You can increase the time schedule based on this criterion up to one time every week. You must stick to this schedule, even on weekends. You can alter the time you go to bed a little, so long as you adhere to the total hours in bed. For example, if you have to get up at 6 a.m. every day for work but want to sleep in until 8 a.m. on the weekend, you would also need to stay up two hours later on Friday night so the total time spent in bed doesn't change from the schedule during the week. Even though it's tempting, don't take a nap during the day. Continue this progression until you arrive at your goal—that is, the ideal number of sleep hours that's best for you.

- If you haven't fallen asleep in about 15 minutes, get out of bed. Leave the bedroom and do something that relaxes you. When you feel like trying to go to sleep again, go back to the bedroom. Whatever you choose to do to relax, do it in the dimmest light possible to avoid triggering the waking part of your circadian rhythm with bright light. I also suggest that you install nightlights so that you don't have to turn lights on to see where you're going. Repeat the getting out of bed cycle as often as necessary.

- If you wake up during the night, do your best not to get upset or worry about it—anxiety over wakefulness will just arouse your brain further. Remind yourself that this is a part of a normal sleep pattern; just try to relax and go back to sleep. If something woke you up, such as the need to go to the bathroom, take care of it and go back to bed. The same recommendation for leaving the bed applies as above if you are not able to go back to sleep within about 15 minutes.

By following this regimen for six to eight weeks, you can expect results similar to those studies that compared this method to the use of prescription sleep medication. You'll avoid the expense, side effects, and potential dependency issues of sleep drugs.

At the end of your sleep behavior therapy period, stick with the step 1 recommendations. They're good habits that will help perpetuate better sleep regardless of your circumstances. You may still sometimes have trouble falling asleep or getting back to sleep if you wake up. If you haven't fallen asleep or gone back to sleep after 30 minutes, get out of bed and do something relaxing, just as you did during step 2.

Your efforts will be worth it. Pleasant dreams!

CHAPTER 14
HAPPINESS AND STRESS CONTROL

W HILE PROPER NUTRITION AND exercise, along with a good night's sleep, are vital to health and fitness, your path to better health and fitness is not complete if you're not as happy and content as you could be. Let's be honest: we all face obstacles in attempting to achieve this, no matter how good our lives may seem to the outside world. For some, these hurdles are insidious, everyday obstacles. For others, the obstacles are steep and painful. Any obstacle to your happiness will create stress in your life—it's just a matter of degree. You can't eliminate stress from your life totally, but you can change your focus. The real enemy isn't stress; it's unhappiness.

I think we all know that too much stress is unhealthy, and I certainly don't need to quote research studies of the health effects of stress to support that claim. What's less obvious, however, is that not all stress is created equal. Obviously, losing your job is significantly more stressful than missing the start of the movie, but that's not the inequality I mean. Different types of stress have different health effects, based in large part on how we view ourselves.

Research tells us that the health of people who view themselves as generally happy is affected by stress less than those who view themselves as generally unhappy. An important distinction here is that this doesn't imply happier people have less stress and generally unhappy people have more stress. The difference is purely based on how the stress affects happy versus unhappy people.

In a study published in the *Proceedings of the National Academy of Sciences* in England, participants were questioned about how often they were happy during the day. The study group ended up recording a variety of happiness levels; some were never happy, some were occasionally happy, and some were happy most of the time. In light of these responses, the researchers looked at levels of the stress hormone cortisol and a marker of inflammation called fibrinogen. Fibrinogen can be elevated when the harmful substances of breakdown aren't balanced by the healing substances of repair. In this study, levels of cortisol were 32 percent lower in people who reported more happy moments. You might expect that people who were happy more often would also have lower levels of fibrinogen in their blood, and this indeed was the case.

The surprising results on the fibrinogen testing, however, came when fibrinogen levels during stress were measured. These results demonstrated that happy people had lower levels of fibrinogen even when under psychological stress. In other words, stress appeared to have *less* of a physical effect on people who were happier. We're all going to experience stress—it's unavoidable. The secret to ensuring that it doesn't negatively affect your health is to be happy most of the time.

This sounds simple, but of course, being happy isn't always that easy. I don't have the secret to happiness, and I can't promise to make you happy, but I can point out some areas that we can all work on. These are areas where human experience and clinical research suggest that you can achieve success in the attainment of greater happiness.

As a physician, I know that sometimes, feelings of deep unhappiness or overwhelming stress are signs of serious problems that require professional care beyond what I can offer in this book. The same goes for problems of substance abuse. If you feel that your unhappiness, feelings of stress, or use of alcohol or drugs are overwhelming your daily life, I urge you to talk to your doctor. Help is available, even if you think your problems are beyond help.

MEANING AND PURPOSE

You can never really achieve lasting happiness if your life doesn't have a source of meaning and purpose. For millennia, human beings have wondered why we are here and whether what we do really matters. Do our lives and their events exist in a vacuum? Does our life relate to some larger whole we're not privy to? In the modern-day world, we still wonder about these things. What do you believe are the answers to these questions? Does what we do matter, or are our life events just a series of vanishing milestones? My belief is that what we do *does* matter, both to ourselves and to the greater whole. What, seriously, is the alternative? To believe that nothing matters simply generates unhappiness and feelings of helplessness and despondency—none of which are helpful or healthful. If you believe that what we do in life matters, then the starting point for everything else is a belief in a higher power. That higher power is not you.

Let me be perfectly clear. I am not telling you where or how to do this. What I am saying is that you need to find a way to give your life meaning and purpose. I believe this means connecting with a higher power in a meaningful way.

Even in remote and underdeveloped civilizations, there has always been a sense that there is something more to this world than meets the eye. Virtually every society in the world has some sort of spiritual belief. The beliefs themselves may be very different, but they have a central theme at their core. This theme essentially revolves around explaining why things are the way they are and what your place in the world is. It usually involves what you must do to be at peace, to be in your proper place in the big picture of the universe. In other words, spiritual belief can be a guide to finding meaning and purpose in your life. This seems to be a universal human need. Seeking meaning and purpose is vital to your well-being. It is fuel for your soul.

When life's meaning is hard to grasp, people may turn to other ways try to feed their soul: alcohol, drugs, money, or power. Odd as it may sound, this reminds me of our annual trek to the pet store to allow our family dog to pick out a birthday present. He will sniff around the toys, but invariably latches onto the "it" dog toy of the moment. Within a few days, however, the toy is chewed through and gone. That's what alcohol, drugs, money, power, and other substitutes for happiness are like. They become our human version of chew toys, things that provide temporary satisfaction but no long-term peace of mind. In the end, these things are poor replacements that can't satisfy our basic need for meaning and purpose.

In addition to looking at the search for meaning in human societies, we can look at it in the anatomical sense by focusing on the structure and function of the brain. Researchers have shown, using brain imaging studies, that certain parts of the brain are activated by different stimuli. When the stimuli involve spirituality, spiritual thoughts create definable patterns of brain activity. The imaging seems to suggest that we're constructed to seek meaning. I don't think this is due to chance. I believe that we are made to seek meaning and purpose—in fact, this is a necessary function to fully realize a fundamental human need.

COMPANIONSHIP

Companionship, another fundamental human need, leads to greater happiness and therefore reduces the harmful effects of stress. The benefit of companionship has been evident for a long time in the study of human development. One example is a famous study of children in an orphanage. The children who were held more often by nurses grew more and were healthier than those who weren't held. A more modern example is that of kids whose families often eat dinner together. The kids in these families generally fare better than those whose families don't eat dinner together. The children who spend dinner time with their families do better in school and are less likely to be obese.

The benefits of companionship are lifelong. Abundant research shows that supportive relationships reduce illness and prolong life. This is especially true in a loving relationship with a spouse. I think we all know of cases where the surviving spouse fades quickly after the death of a loving partner. This isn't to say that your spouse is responsible for your happiness. You're still responsible for your own happiness, but we're certainly better able to weather life's storms when we have strong bonds of companionship. In a good relationship, marriage, or friendship, your own happiness is often much easier to achieve. The emotional investment to ensure the benefit from strong relationships—especially close relationships, such as your marriage—is, without question, worthwhile.

Although a spouse or life partner can provide you with the caring and supportive companionship that is so vital to us all, other relationships—friends, family members, significant others—can be equally important. Think back to some of the best moments of your life. How many of those moments involve you by yourself? Chances are, it's the shared moments that bring the biggest smile to your face. When you receive great news, is your next thought to share it with someone or to go to your room and celebrate alone? Have you ever been on a trip and have the adventure lose its luster because you weren't able to experience it with a certain someone? We are wired to be with others.

In our busy society, the biggest obstacle to nurturing valuable relationships is often finding the time to make the effort. We all get caught up in our daily responsibilities and routines, and before we know it, little energy is left for our relationships. Even a little time is better than none, though. You don't have to have a grand plan or schedule an outing to nurture a relationship. Even a short phone conversation, or sending a text to let someone know you're thinking about him or her, can make a positive difference to the bond. If you really want to make your doctor happy, take a walk or go to the gym with a friend or loved one. Simply put, make spending time with those who are close to you a priority.

Companionship can also come in a less personal setting. Look around your community and you will see bowling leagues, car clubs, garden clubs, recreational sports teams, volunteer organizations, church groups, book clubs, and countless other ways that people get together. These activities provide great avenues to pursue our interests and to meet others who share those interests. Getting out and being involved with the community is good for everyone, but it's especially important if you're retired or live alone. People who are socially isolated are known to have higher rates of illness, including a substantially higher risk for developing dementia. Elvis was right in "Heartbreak Hotel" when he sang, "I'm so lonely I could die." Not surprisingly, isolation is also associated with higher levels of unhappiness. Social isolation is literally a killer. Find something or someone whose company you enjoy and get involved if you are not doing so already.

Another level of companionship that has been shown to increase human happiness is interaction with animals. In one study conducted in 1980, pet owners who had a heart attack had higher survival rates after one year than those who didn't own a pet. Subsequent studies have shown that pet owners tend to have lower blood pressure, less loneliness, and lower cholesterol. They are also happier overall. Pet therapy programs that bring animals into nursing homes and hospitals have been shown to promote a greater sense of well-being in patients.

I've had a number of patients who have shown substantial improvements in their health and happiness after adopting a pet. It's not entirely clear why the benefits of pet ownership are so pronounced, but if you have ever had your dog enthusiastically greet you when you get home, or petted a purring cat, you probably inherently relate to why this would be true. I understand that having a pet isn't for everyone; and it's not for every circumstance. Pets certainly don't replace the need for human companionship, but they can be a potential source of happiness in your life.

NOTICE AND APPRECIATE: MINDFULNESS

One more pillar supports the structure of your happiness: taking notice and appreciating the simple things in the world around you. In other words, being mindful.

We tend to be so busy and focused on our tasks that we miss much of what goes on around us. We rush from errand to errand, place to place. We are so intent on the destination that we miss the beauty of the journey.

Happiness isn't about success or hyped-up super arousal; it is much more peaceful than that. Happiness is about being content or satisfied with your life, having the courage to change the things you want to change and taking pleasure in the simple things. Sometimes we just need to stop, notice, and appreciate what we already have in our lives.

We must recognize that there is a rhythm to our existence. This rhythm includes work, but it also includes relaxation. It includes doing, but it also includes thinking and observing. It lets us see that the world does not revolve around us. No matter what we didn't get accomplished today, the sun, as Annie sings, will always come out tomorrow.

Do you remember the song "Cat's in the Cradle" by Harry Chapin? The song is essentially about a boy's growing up from his father's perspective. The father was a loving man but was so busy with work that he missed many opportunities to be involved in his son's life. The boy wasn't upset by this, but rather wanted to emulate his father. "I'm going to be just like him," he says. At the end of the song, the father is old, and the boy has grown up. The father calls his son and says he wants to see him. His son, now with responsibilities of his own, is too busy to see his father. "He grew up just like me," the father ruefully concludes. Both of them end up missing out on the treasure of their relationship. This message applies to us all, in all relationships and situations. Take a look at your life to see if you are missing any treasure. Don't find yourself looking back with regret at the moments you missed out on. Figure out what is important to you before it's too late and notice and appreciate those things fully.

Notice the natural beauty around you. It's everywhere, if you look for it. The first daffodils or wildflowers emerging in the springtime or the turn of fall foliage can be uplifting if you stop to notice them and appreciate their beauty. It can be captivating to watch rain coming down on your car from one isolated cloud on an otherwise sunny day (my kids made fun of me for being enamored with that one day). I'm not suggesting that you go overboard with this, but perspective can be very helpful. Gary

Larson illustrated perspective beautifully in a *Far Side* cartoon. It shows an artist with a beautiful painting of a bird on his canvas. When you look beyond the artist's easel, however, the full scene is revealed. The bird is, in fact, sitting on trash in a garbage dump. It all depends on what you choose to see.

The relevance of perspective and what you choose to see was shown brilliantly demonstrated in 1999 by the famous invisible gorilla experiment conducted by Daniel Simons of the University of Illinois and Christopher Chabris of Harvard. They asked a group of students to watch a recording of a basketball game, with the express instruction to count the number of passes that occurred between one side. During the recording, a person in a gorilla outfit can be seen walking onto the basketball court for a full nine seconds before leaving the court, weaving in and out between the players and even stopping to thump its chest. When the viewers were quizzed about how many passes they counted in the recording, fewer than half of them saw the gorilla! They were so focused on counting the basketball passes that their brain didn't register what was right in front of them.

The same thing happens to us all the time. We can be so busy being busy that we forget to notice and appreciate the beauty in everyday life. And yet, if you shift your perspective, you might be surprised at just how much there already is in your life to be grateful for and just how happy you could choose to be. As Stephen Covey says, "Happiness, like unhappiness, is a proactive choice."

WHAT ABOUT STRESS?

When we seek to establish meaning and purpose in our lives, to foster companionship, and to take notice and appreciate the simple things, we increase our ability to handle the inevitable stresses that come our way. To understand why, let's look more closely at what stress actually is, how it affects your body, and how you can maximize your body's defense against it.

Stress is your body's reaction to any sort of change—positive or negative—that requires a physical, mental, or emotional adjustment or response. In stressful situations that could be harmful, your body reacts with its in-built "fight-or-flight" response. The response alerts you to danger and is designed to keep you safe. In the same way that a rabbit's physiology will change when it sees a fox, our physiology also changes in the face of danger. Our heart rate goes up, we breathe faster, more blood goes to the brain and muscles and less blood goes to the digestive tract, and our muscles become tense and ready for action. However, in the modern world, we no longer have to battle with cave lions or run from mammoths, so we only rarely confront a genuine fight-or-flight situation. Unfortunately, the response is still triggered as a result of much more familiar worldly demands.

Stress can be divided into acute and chronic types. Acute types of stress are short-acting stresses, such as being late to work because you were caught in traffic. Chronic stresses are prolonged and can be things like divorce or a bad family relationship, losing or hating your job, or a death or illness in the family. Chronic stresses are difficult to alleviate—caring for a dying parent, for instance, can last for a long time and usually only gets more stressful as time goes by. Often nothing can be done. In these difficult situations, spirituality and good relationships can be particularly valuable for helping you cope. And if you're already suffering from chronic stress, adding acute stress on top of it is the last thing you need.

Even isolated, everyday acute stresses, however, can act like chronic stress on the body if they are part of the way you relate to the world. We can exert a lot more control over acute stress and how it affects us than we can with chronic stress.

How daily life events affect us differs widely from person to person—clearly individuals respond very differently to the same stressful situations. Some people thrive on and enjoy situations that might make another person cringe. Public speaking comes to mind. An extroverted person may love the chance to give a talk; a shy person may dread it. Some things, such as an unexpected change in your schedule, may be stressful to you in one frame of mind, but in another frame of mind, don't bother you at all. This has a lot to do with your perspective.

Not all stress is a result of something bad. Having a new baby or getting a promotion are positive things that can cause stress. Sometimes we see things as stressful or not stressful based on our perception of our ability to cope with the situation. You may recognize this when you feel stressed about something at night or when you're tired from a long day. After a good night's sleep, the same problem can seem much less overwhelming. Stress can also be a useful tool. It can provide motivation for getting something done. In moderate amounts, it can improve performance.

Anything that causes stress is called a stressor. Your personal stressors will change, based on all of the variables above, but identifying them can be a good start to minimizing their impact. You can also reduce your stress levels if you can identify the things and situations that put you in the frame of mind where stressors are magnified. Many of my patients benefit from making a list of the things that create stress in their life and the things that contribute to magnifying that stress. Awareness of the obvious and not-so-obvious issues can really help you manage stress appropriately.

Managing stress isn't easy—I know I can use all the help I can get. Over the years, I've put together some ideas that have helped a lot of my patients. These day-to-day ideas are most effective if you also attend to the other aspects of your life—finding meaning and purpose, finding companionship, finding beauty in the everyday. Read through them with an open mind—I hope you will find ideas that could work for you.

FOR THE BODY

In addition to every other benefit of exercise I've already discussed, exercise is a wonderful stress-reducing tool. (You didn't think I'd miss an opportunity to further promote its good effects, did you?) Not only does exercise help reduce stress, but many studies indicate that it helps relieve depression and anxiety as well. You will be hard-pressed to remember a time when you didn't feel mentally better after exercise than you did before exercise.

- Massage is a great way to relax and unwind. In addition to how good it makes you feel, studies suggest that massage has some demonstrable health benefits. Treat yourself to a massage when you can. If you have never had a massage, don't underestimate how much relaxation it provides.

- Consider a regular meditation practice as a way to further release your stresses. Meditation comes in many forms, but in general, it works by briefly focusing your attention on a single point of thought or awareness; other concerns then fade away or are put into perspective. You don't need to be a yogi or maharishi to do this—in fact, just about anyone can learn the basic meditation techniques quickly and on their own. Sometimes just closing the door for a few minutes and freeing your mind can do wonders. Numerous studies have shown that transcendental meditation (TM) helps create a state of restful alertness that can reduce stress, anxiety, and fatigue. It has also been shown to help lower cortisol levels and reduce high blood pressure.

- Yoga and tai chi are not only great core exercises, but they are also great for calming the mind.

- Directed muscle relaxation, also known as progressive muscle relaxation, is a technique that you can use at home. While sitting or reclining comfortably, start by clenching the muscles of your toes. Then consciously relax those same muscles. Do the same for the muscles of your feet, then your lower legs, and progress your way up your body until you get to the muscles in your forehead. This takes just a couple of minutes and produces good results.

- Getting enough sleep will also help you cope with stress constructively.

FOR THE MIND

- Preparation is key to stress reduction. As much as you can, prepare for your day the night before. Set out your clothes, have your lunch ready to pack, set out anything you have to remember to take the next day. The same concept applies to planning ahead. If you're going to take a long drive today, make sure you filled the gas tank yesterday. Try to set up contingency plans ahead of time in case you run into difficulties. For example, make sure you know the location of a spare set of car keys and have an extra house key stored at a trusted neighbor's home.

- Over-committing is a major cause of stress. Be willing to say no. It's OK, really. If you don't have the time, energy, or desire for an optional activity, you probably shouldn't do it. This is a hard but necessary skill to master.

- Give yourself 15 minutes more than you think you need. This could apply to getting up in the morning or driving to an appointment or meeting. Getting there a couple of minutes early and having a moment to relax is always preferable to running late.

- Turn off your phone, computer, smart phone, e-mail, or whatever else keeps you from getting some uninterrupted time. Everything will still be there when you plug back in.

- Doing something good for someone else almost always makes you feel better. Consider what you could do to make someone else's life a little easier today. Think about how you could do good on a regular basis, perhaps through regular volunteer work.

- Accept that there are things and people we simply cannot change. Trying to do so will only create more stress. The hard part sometimes is accepting the fact that we can't change the situation. I imagine we can all think of someone or something in our life that this applies to. If you can't change it, let it go—it's not worth it.

- Don't put things off that you can get done now. I'm certainly guilty of procrastination myself, but I can also tell you from personal experience that it's stressful. If you do what you need to do now, you won't have to deal with it later, at a time when your stress levels might be even higher. This is not to say that if you're already feeling overwhelmed, you need to get mundane things done now. At the end of a long day, sometimes the dishes can wait until tomorrow. They're not going anywhere. On the other hand, if you had plenty of opportunity to get them done and you didn't, a sink full of dirty dishes the next morning may seem like even more of a burden. Along this same line, if you have to do something today that you find stressful, try to do it early in the day. Get it over with so you can be more productive and relaxed the rest of the day.

- For day-to-day stresses, try to put things in perspective. Will something that is stressing you now really make your life different a year from now? How many day-to-day stresses five years ago made your life different today?

- Don't just read through this list and think that some of these things make sense. Put them into practice where they apply to you.

I understand many of the thoughts in this chapter are easier said than done, but they are all doable, even if they take a bit of effort. My hope is that some of the thoughts will help you shift your perspective so you can increase your happiness and decrease your stress.

CHAPTER 15
ACHIEVING SUCCESS

B ECOMING A FIT AND healthy version of you doesn't mean you have to change who you are. It means you need to decide what an energetic, healthy, happy life is worth to you and then consciously choose that path. No one expects you to be perfect. But the fact remains, the more action you take to improve your health and the more recommendations you embrace from this book, the better your odds for achieving your goals. It also follows that the more often you take action and follow the recommendations, the better the outcome and the quicker you will notice the positive effects of a fit and healthy lifestyle.

Be patient with yourself. Don't expect that you will pick up all of the recommendations here straightaway and run with them all. That's unrealistic. As soon as you fall short of your impossibly high expectations, you may simply quit—and that's the worst thing you can do. Start by adopting one or two of the recommendations—the ones that seem to make the most sense to you or are easiest to do—and add more gradually.

Remember Russ's story from the beginning of the book? Russ simply decided one day that he needed to improve his health and his life. He started with just one easy step: eliminating sugary soft drinks from his diet. If you want to improve your health, start with something that seems particularly doable to you, or something that inspires you. Step by step, you will gain confidence in yourself and gather the positive momentum that can help you through the more involved stages.

YOU+ ACTION PLAN

Taking action, no matter what it is, is how the YOU+ plan can help you become healthier and happier. The list of critical steps to take is helpful, but remember: not every step may be right for you right now. Choose what works for you today; the other steps will fall into place over time.

THE MOST IMPORTANT STEP IS THE FIRST STEP:

1. Commit to your health and fitness once and for all. No more excuses—today is the day you change your life.

FOOD AND DRINK STEPS:

2. Eat three meals a day.

3. Use the proper ratio for your food. Your protein portions should be roughly the size of your hand. The total of all starches (carbohydrates) should also be roughly the size of your hand. For people who want to lose weight quickly, or for people who have a hard time losing weight, the ratio of protein to starch should be modified to cut back on the starch. In that case, the protein portion should be the size of your whole hand, and the starch portion should be roughly the size of your palm. The ratio becomes 2:1, or roughly twice as much protein as starch.

4. For second helpings, wait at least 20 minutes from the time you begin eating your meal; keep the size ratio the same, even if the amount you choose is smaller. (Check back to Chapter 5 for details on how to achieve the proper ratios.)

5. Starches include bread, pasta, rolls, rice, potatoes, tortillas, couscous, and similar foods. Aim for whole grains or whole foods whenever possible. Sweets count as starches and should be limited.

6. For protein, choose primarily skinless poultry or fish; lean pork and beef should be less than one-third of your protein intake in any particular week. Avoid processed meat. All lean protein can be baked, sautéed, broiled, boiled, or grilled. Dairy items and eggs count as a protein; three servings of dairy daily are recommended. Nuts count as a protein source. If you don't eat animal foods, think of beans as a protein if they're the main part of a meal. If you do eat animal foods or if the beans are a side dish, think of them as a vegetable.

7. Fruits and vegetables are completely free in the YOU+ eating plan; eat at least one fruit and/or vegetable at every meal.

8. Men should consume about 100 ounces of fluid each day; women need about 72 ounces each day. Your fluids should come mostly from water, tea (iced or hot), coffee, and milk.

9. Once a week, enjoy a half-day cheat. During that time, splurge and eat something that you wouldn't regularly consume on the YOU+ eating plan, such as ice cream or pizza.

10. The only dietary supplements you need to take (outside of the nutrient timing supplements discussed in Chapter 12) are omega-3 fatty acids, commonly found in fish oil, vitamin D, and glutamine. Take a fish oil supplement containing at least 500 mg of EPA/DHA on days you don't eat fish. Vitamin D supplement amounts will depend on a blood test result, but most people need at least 1,000 units daily. Take 5 grams of glutamine daily.

EXERCISE STEPS:

11. Ideally, join a gym.

12. Work out with resistance training (strength training) three times a week, as detailed in Chapter 10. To help you properly plan and track your workouts, use the YOU+ app or website.

13. Incorporate aerobic (cardio) exercise into your workout program three times a week for 20 to 30 minutes, as detailed in chapters 9 and 10. Vary the activity and intensity of activity for maximum enjoyment and improvement.

14. If it's more convenient for you to complete your strength and aerobic training in one session, do your aerobic activity *after* your strength training.

15. Warm up with a few minutes of aerobic activity before any exercise routine, and run through the full range of motions you are about to perform, as detailed in Chapter 11.

16. After your work out, cool down with passive or static stretches to elongate the muscles and help promote maximal recovery.

17. The best time to exercise is when you can exercise. Any time is better than no time.

18. Include core training and strength in your exercise schedule for just a few minutes three times weekly (see Chapter 11). Strong core muscles give you greater mobility, improve your posture, and help to prevent injury and pain.

19. Balance can be improved by three simple exercises that can be done anywhere—see Chapter 11.

20. To improve your workout results, promote leanness, and improve post-workout repair, use supplements containing branched chain amino acids (BCAAs) and whey protein.

21. Take a total of 3 to 5 grams (3,000 to 5,000 milligrams) of BCAAs with plain water a few minutes before starting exercise. The BCAAs you choose should contain at least 50 percent leucine in capsule form.

22. Following or during aerobic activity, rehydrate by drinking at least 16 ounces of water. Don't drink sports drinks before or after a workout; the extra calories may cancel out all your effort.

23. Following strength training or active aerobic training, mix 20 to 25 grams of whey protein powder with around 10 grams of carbohydrate from a rapidly absorbing source, such as Gatorade powder. Add about 12 ounces of water, shake, and drink. Drink the whey protein immediately after working out, or no later than one hour afterward.

HEALTH AND MOTIVATION STEPS:

24. Aim to get at least seven hours of good quality sleep every night.

25. Health and fitness can be a fun journey. To help with your enjoyment and motivation, find a training partner.

26. Celebrate successes, laugh off setbacks, and start afresh tomorrow. Being happy can counteract the effects of stress.

27. Relish how good you feel now that you have finally taken charge of your health and fitness. Commit to living life to the fullest.

Successfully living a fit and healthy lifestyle is easier said than done. But, as the saying goes, nothing in life worth having is easy. Part of the challenge is having the right knowledge so you can avoid wasted time and effort—that's what this book and the YOU+ app and website are for.

But right knowledge is just part of the equation. The other part is right action. It doesn't matter if you know what to do but still don't do it. If you're currently not eating any of the right foods and doing zero exercise or activity, then the best way to succeed is to make gradual, incremental modifications. That way, you can implement long-term, meaningful change and enjoy the vibrant health and vitality you deserve.

Very few people can go from zero to hero in one fluid step. It's all too easy to fall at the first hurdle and give up. Change isn't an overnight affair. It's not a linear process. You will make progress and then fall back—this is normal. Remember: "Rome wasn't built in a day." When you make incremental changes to your behavior, it helps to accept from the outset that some days will be better than others. But I promise you this: you will never lose so long as you never give up. If you commit to the YOU+ program and persevere past the times you want to give up, then you *will* achieve your goals. You only guarantee your failure by not trying.

MAKING THE DECISION TO CHANGE

Deciding to make fitness a part of your life isn't just an intellectual decision. It's an emotional decision as well. If it were purely intellectual, wouldn't everyone do it? Wouldn't everyone decide to feel better, achieve a healthy weight, and be less susceptible to cancer, heart disease, joint pain, and the myriad of other complaints we have been talking about?

As you journey toward health, there will be naysayers. Some people will doubt your commitment or ability to follow the YOU+ plan. Others will discourage you because your decision to change makes them uncomfortably aware of their own lack of fitness. It's quite likely that the people who are discouraging or negative about your change of lifestyle are those close to you. Their lack of support can be hurtful. Remember that you are doing all of this for your own health and well-being—you deserve to live a better life, no matter what others say.

Sometimes other people will try to discourage you by pointing to someone who lives a decidedly unhealthy lifestyle but still appears to be doing pretty well. They might remind you about your old Uncle George, who smoked two packs of cigarettes a day and is still alive at age 95. They conveniently forget about your Uncle Fred, who smoked two packs a day and died of a heart attack when he was 50. You could put on a blindfold and walk across a busy freeway, and you *might* actually make it in one piece. But that still doesn't make it a good idea! Conversely, someone might mention a person who did all the right health things and still got cancer or heart disease. Of course, even fit people with a good lifestyle become sick with serious diseases, but they tilt the odds against disease in their favor by being healthy—and if they do get sick, being healthy otherwise tilts the odds in favor of recovery and survival.

In the end, a healthy lifestyle simply comes down to improving your odds as best you can. It may be true that someone with an unhealthy lifestyle stays healthy, or someone with a healthy lifestyle becomes ill, but that defies the odds. Since, in a way, you're betting your life on the decisions you make, shouldn't you get the best odds you can? Even the best bets don't pan out 100 percent of the time. There are always exceptions to every rule, but the smart bet is on the rule.

The emotional component of the fitness decision is often the hardest part to crack. For most people, the catalyst for genuine change comes down to the simple realization that they just need to do it. No more sitting on the sidelines or dabbling on the edges—the time has come to embrace fitness once and for all.

Often this starts with a conscious shifting of priorities. Someone who decides to get fit has usually found that something important to him or her is the impetus. Perhaps it's as simple as not wanting to buy the bigger clothes, but often it's a personal reason, such as wanting more energy to play with the kids, having a health scare, or the dawning realization that health isn't a birthright. Like most things in life worth having, health must be earned.

THINGS THAT GET IN THE WAY

To fully embrace a healthy lifestyle, you may need to address the things that can get in your way. Near the top of the list is the tendency to put off getting fit until later. It's not that you lack interest in getting healthy; it's just that it seems there are always other things you have to do first. Maybe it's when you get that promotion or when you reach retirement, or, maybe it's after the kids start school or leave home. My patients usually start these explanations with "If only . . ." They tell me, for example, "If only my spouse would . . ." or, "If only I hadn't let myself get this far out of shape . . . " Forget about "if only." We're all responsible for ourselves; it's up to us to make the changes we desire. We all have the power to choose. We all make our own decisions concerning how we may live. Exerting control over these decisions is uplifting and powerful—it can turn any negative into a positive.

I often hear from my patients that fitness choices are completely guided by one spouse or the other. The bottom line is that your spouse doesn't put the fork into your mouth; you decide what goes in there. Nothing dictates that you can't do the grocery shopping once in a while. Nothing says that you can't order what you want when you go to a restaurant. Nothing says that you can't decide to exercise instead of watching something on

TV that doesn't even interest you. Take responsibility for yourself and the decisions you make. Procrastination and postponing are good strategies if you want to let things slip away from you, but I don't recommend that.

Once you start, don't take your eye off the ball. We have so many toys and gadgets to occupy our time and infinite ways to entertain ourselves, so it's easy to become distracted from the really important stuff.

When I was a little boy, I went on a fishing trip with my father and a friend of his. My dad and I weren't exactly outdoorsmen, but this guy was a true aficionado of the outdoor life. We weren't planning to do anything fancy—we mostly just wanted to learn how to catch some small pan fish. When we arrived at the lake, we set up on the shore. I was eager to learn some fishing secrets from my dad's friend. What he did next, however, didn't exactly match with the image of the great outdoorsman I had in mind. He took out a can of corn, opened it, and threw some of the kernels into the water. This, it turned out, was the fishing secret. The water came alive with fish streaming to the surface to feast on the meal he had thrown to them. The next thing I knew, I had corn kernels on my hook. I cast my line into the water and found that the fish were so eager to devour the corn that they went for the kernels attached to my fishing pole. We had a good time and caught a lot of fish.

So what are the corn kernels in your life? What distractions do you devour so unthinkingly that they take you away from what you know you should do? Don't let these things be attached to a life-robbing hook.

The granddaddy of all things that get in the way of living a fit life is the idea that you don't have time for it. I absolutely believe that you are very busy. I absolutely do not believe that you have too little time to be fit. It's simply a matter of making fitness a priority. Listen, I understand busy. As a full-time physician with a family, I get it. I know that time is in short supply. Given this reality, if something is important enough to you, you will find time for it. If you have an important event tomorrow and you have to pick up your clothes from the dry cleaner before they close today, you will find a way to get there. If there's something that's fun for you and that you enjoy doing, you will likely find a way to make time for it. If you receive a free spa treatment or tickets to the big game, you probably will find time to go. Maybe the real issue is that deep down, you don't want to find the time, and lack of time is a handy excuse. It's also possible that you've tried to get fit in the past but found that your efforts weren't as successful or enjoyable as you had hoped. The perceived lack of enjoyment and success can be a major stumbling block. I can't make you enjoy becoming fit and healthy, but I can assure you that with the YOU+ plan, your fitness efforts will feel considerably better, and you will get much more out of them. When you see your work paying off and even start to enjoy it, you are much more likely to stick to the plan.

WHAT OTHERS HAVE FOUND HELPFUL

Some people are inspired by looking at fitness as a competition with themselves. If you are a goal-oriented person, comparing what you can do now to get in shape versus what you could do when you started can be a great motivator. Whether it's flexibility, balance, endurance, strength, or eating right, setting and achieving milestones for yourself can be a great motivator. Aim for milestones that are realistic and attainable—and incremental. Setting a major fitness goal that is far out in the future can be a mistake because you won't have much feedback in the short term to keep you going. By setting incremental benchmarks along the way, you give yourself positive reinforcement as you pass each one toward your ultimate goal.

It doesn't matter what your starting point is; what matters is the progress you make from that point forward. Don't be discouraged if you have to start from a de-conditioned low point. I have had patients who could barely manage five minutes on a treadmill at the start of their fitness program and could only increase their time by a minute every week or two. But small improvements add up—after six months, these patients were up to half an hour at a time on the treadmill and had added strength training as well. They were substantially fitter than when they started, and it showed in their weight and their ability to get through the activities of daily living more easily.

Some of my patients begin their fitness program with lofty goals of running a marathon, a training regimen that can take over a year. They soon realize, however, that in the meantime, running in shorter local races, such as a 5K charity event, is a lot of fun. Competing in the shorter races gives them the inspiration to stick with the larger goal.

Wherever you are on your journey to fitness, the only person you should compare yourself to is the one you see when you look in the mirror. Advancing your own health and happiness is the only benchmark that matters.

Whatever your fitness goal, you will find that varying your training and experimenting with new techniques helps keep life interesting and improves results. Some aspects of the YOU+ program, such as the cheat day on your eating plan and the emphasis on frequently changing up your workout, let you achieve the variety that helps keep you on track. Finding a training partner is also very helpful. Consider teaming up with someone with similar goals so you can transition to a fit lifestyle together. Maybe a friend or coworker is struggling with the same issues as you. Sharing your goals openly with someone supportive can be very helpful.

Even though I already have a strong commitment to a fit lifestyle and counsel others on the subject, I still find it helpful to get support from my workout pals. They help me stay true to the fit lifestyle I enjoy and also keep me from becoming complacent or bored. We support each other with humor; we always have a good laugh when we are together. We also support each other with understanding and encouragement. When one of us loses focus, the others will tell him to go get a drink from the "fountain of positive thinking." That's what we call the water fountain when someone needs to reset their point of view in a more positive direction.

Whether you work out with someone else, a group, or by yourself, find your own version of the fountain of positive thinking. On those days when you just aren't compelled to exercise, even though you know how important it is and how much you will benefit from it, positive thinking is a valuable tool. The support of others can help you stay positive and motivate you to get to the gym. In the end, however, you are still ultimately responsible for you. The gains you make in your fitness are your own.

The element of habit plays a big role in your exercise program. Simply put, fitness needs to be something that you do as part of your normal routine. This isn't as easy a habit to develop as munching junk food while watching TV or stopping for a not-so-healthy muffin on the way to work. But, like any habit, repetition is key—stick with it.

No matter what I've told you about how great you will eventually feel, you may find that when you first start working out, you just plain don't like it. Give it the six introductory weeks outlined in Chapter 8. For those six weeks, fight through any dislike and do what you know you need to do—even if you don't want to. Making the effort for six weeks allows your body to detox from the negative effects of a bad diet and low activity levels.

After detoxing, healthy habits will be much easier to maintain. By week six—quite probably sooner—you'll begin to notice different ways your effort is paying off. You'll reach a point where you don't feel as well if you skip a few days of your fitness plan.

As the old saying goes, "A journey of a thousand miles begins with a single step." Taking the first step is the hardest part of your fitness journey. What gets you to take that first step will be unique to you. Find what drives you. What led you to pick up this book in the first place? Is it overall health, weight loss, longevity, vigor, or something else? Maybe you simply don't want to buy the larger size of clothes. Whatever it is, grab the bull by the horns and get to it.

Congratulations for reading this book! You've now taken the critical first step. By doing so, you've already put yourself in the top percentile of people who take their health and well-being seriously. The benefits of vibrant health, energy, and vitality are disproportionately high for the relatively small amount of effort you invest. Just think about it for a moment. A week has 168 hours. If you use just three of those hours during the week to exercise regularly, you'll find that the remaining 165 hours are transformed in a variety of ways. Those aches and pains you've convinced yourself are just part of getting older will disappear or, at least, will diminish. That extra weight you couldn't seem to lose will melt away, and you will unleash a reservoir of energy you didn't think possible. You will greatly reduce your risk of every possible serious illness—from heart disease to cancer and everything else in between. And, perhaps best of all, you'll feel like a million dollars. Don't put your health and well-being off for another moment. Enjoy the journey and reap the rewards.

ACKNOWLEDGEMENTS

A book is definitely a team effort, and there are a number of people who I am grateful to for their help, influence, and contributions to this project.

Sheila Buff, my book doctor and editor, has been instrumental in guiding this project from beginning to end. Her wisdom, experience, and forthrightness have been invaluable and she has made everything better.

I am deeply appreciative to Rod Thomas. Without his belief and dedication to better health for all, this project would never have been possible.

I have learned so much from my patients over the years, and without them, I would have never acquired the knowledge and experience that has shaped my medical practice and passion for health care.

A long list of people have positively influenced my career and direction. You each know the role you have played. Thank you to Kelly Cain, Mark and Mieko Catron, John Acquavella, Jim Slattery, Lynn and Deena Jones, Charlie Hale, Chuck Thal, John Davidson, Gilda Taylor, Barry Highbloom, Erle Taube, and Kim and Brian Bell.

And of course I am grateful to my family. Thank you for your tireless love and support in spite of the late nights and weekends pursuing my passion for health and fitness.

INDEX